Karin Schutt

Ayurveda

The secret of lifelong youth

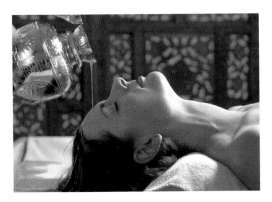

A practical home programme covering:

- eating to suit your constitutional type

- top-to-toe massage

- strength and relaxation exercises

TIME-LIFE BOOKS, AMSTERDAM

Contents

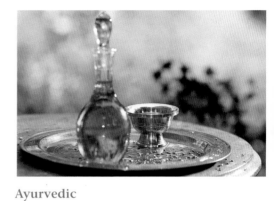

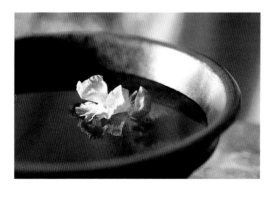

Important

This book provides a modern interpretation of Ayurveda,
specially adapted for use in the West. The purpose of the exercises
and advice is to preserve health, improve general well-being and
prevent illness. The exercises are also suitable for those suffering
from minor, everyday stress-related symptoms, such as anxiety,
tension and fatigue. The advice given in the book is no substitute
for Ayurvedic therapy based on detailed diagnosis and personally
prescribed care, nor can it replace treatment of health problems by
a traditional doctor or a qualified Ayurvedic practitioner.

Foreword

Ayurveda is the oldest known form of healing, more ancient than Chinese medicine, and very much older than Western medicine. The term *Ayurveda* comes from Sanskrit, the religious and philosophical language of ancient India. *Ved* means knowledge or science and *ayu* means daily life or life cycle, representing a doctrine of holistic healing which aims to promote and maintain the total well-being of the individual. This "science of life" embraces both preventive measures and therapeutic procedures, which can be especially effective in the treatment of chronic disorders. As a means of self-help, Ayurveda will enable you to improve your general health and to become more aware of your body's natural needs and how to satisfy them.

Ayurveda – an ancient healing art

My intention in writing this book is to introduce you to Ayurveda and encourage you to follow a path that will lead you to the sources of your physical and spiritual well-being. The Ayurvedic self-help techniques are specially tailored to provide you with a simple system to enable you to achieve lasting health and realize your full potential, by first recovering and then maintaining your natural inner harmony. If you follow the exercises you will find you have increased energy for daily tasks, and feel more at ease with yourself. However, this book cannot perform miracles. It is intended as a guide to help you find your own way to health: your well-being is entirely in your own hands.

Ayurveda today is not practised exactly as it was in India more than three thousand years ago. Over the years it has been adapted to suit changing ways of life. This book presents a version of Ayurveda tailored to meet the needs of readers in the West. The adaptation was only made possible through the help and support of experienced experts in the field. I should therefore like to offer my sincerest thanks to Dr John Switzer, Ayurvedic practitioner and homeopath, and Ms. Merholz, health counsellor at the Maharishi-Ayur-Ved Health Centre at Pöcking/Starnberger See.

The science of life

Karin Schutt

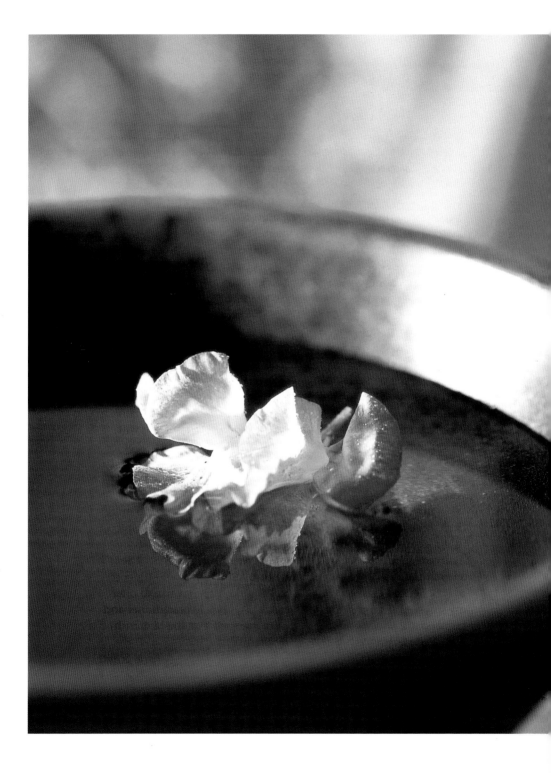

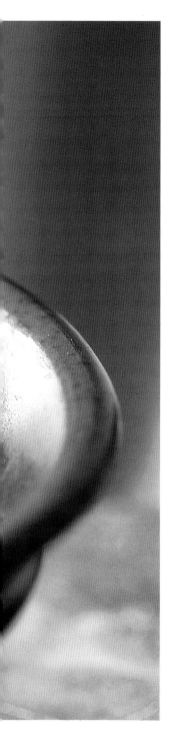

The science of long life

"Ayurveda is concerned with the whole of life: both pain and pleasure are important aspects of this science. This means that, on the one hand, Ayurveda teaches us how to rid ourselves of pain and suffering; on the other hand it teaches us different ways of increasing our enjoyment of life."
Dr Vinod Verma

Adding years to life, adding life to years – this is the essence of Ayurveda, the Indian art of healing. Ayurvedic treatises dating back thousands of years lay down precise instructions on how and by what means each individual can achieve physical and spiritual well-being.
For only when body, mind and soul live in harmony is complete health possible.

What is Ayurveda?

Traditional Indian philosophy and religion provide the intellectual basis of Ayurveda. Built on spiritual foundations, Ayurveda is an extensive doctrine embracing both human health and humanity's relationship with the heavens and the cosmos. The methods of treatment are founded on a multilayered diagnostic process that provide information both about temporary ailments and about an individual's constitutional type.

Health and sickness in Ayurveda

Harmonizing the life energies

The first objective of Ayurvedic therapy is to restore any imbalance between the vital life energies. The next stage is geared towards establishing long-term stability and optimum health. The overriding aim of the whole Ayurvedic system is a long life free from disease and suffering. This aim goes hand-in-hand with the development of intellectual potential through increased awareness and greater respect for the spiritual side of life.

To make sense of Ayurveda you need to give equal attention to both theory and practice. It is just as important to grasp the underlying theory as it is to carry out the practical exercises. With this in mind, do not turn straight to the exercises, but give yourself time to absorb the philosophy and terminology which are further explained in this introductory section of the book. In order to gain a full and deep understanding of this ancient life science you need first to learn about its spiritual basis and familiarize yourself with some of its special language.

Learning to understand

Health means more than the absence of disease

The Indian art of healing is concerned with every sphere of life and the harmonious interaction of them all. The emotions, intellect, body, actions, our general behaviour and the environment in which we live are all interlinked and influence each other. We should neither focus only on, nor ignore, any single one of them. Inspired by this holistic perspective, those who practise Ayurveda attempt to create and maintain a balance between all the components of existence.

Harmony between body, mind and emotions

1 Balance is a central concept of Ayurveda and is synonymous with health. Equilibrium brings with it sensations of inner harmony, contentment and lasting well-being. Once balance is achieved, the individual gains a feeling of wholeness and happiness, a feeling of being at one with the cosmos. Ayurvedic teachings tell us that the healthy person is one whose bodily functions – metabolism, digestion, tissues and elimination – are balanced, and whose mind, soul and senses are in a state of inner peace and contentment.

2 According to Ayurveda, all bodily, mental and spiritual functions are controlled by three vital energies called the doshas. Equilibrium between these three forces is essential for the maintenance of well-being. When the doshas become unbalanced, health suffers.

Interaction between the spheres of life

3 Imbalance occurs when a person continually works against his or her own nature over a prolonged period. It could be the result of an unhealthy or unsuitable diet, an inappropriate lifestyle or behaviour, negative thoughts or emotions, stress or other environmental factors. If balance is not restored and the discord is allowed to continue, health breaks down and the person becomes ill.

**Balancing
the doshas**

4 According to Ayurvedic theory, illness is the outcome of long-term imbalance of the vital forces. The main effect is a damaging build-up of *ama* – toxins and waste products. Ayurvedic therapy aims first and foremost to rid the body of ama, so restoring the equilibrium of the doshas.

Balance and wholeness, doshas and ama. These connections and concepts are crucial to an understanding of Ayurveda. They are explained in more detail in the following chapters.

The theory of the three doshas

The "Tridosha theory" – *tri* meaning three and *dosha* meaning fault or weakness – is at the heart of the Ayurvedic art of healing. The theory states that the mental, spiritual and physical functions of an individual are governed by three vital forces or regulatory principles: *vata*, *pitta* and *kapha*. These three forces combine in each person, in proportions that vary from one person to another. Each of the three doshas is subdivided into five secondary doshas. This precision makes it possible to differentiate exactly between the individual bodily functions and spiritual states, and so reach an accurate diagnosis and prescribe therapy for specific complaints.

**Primary
forces**

In this book, we shall deal only with the three main doshas. It is important to understand that these forces – vata, pitta and kapha – can neither be seen nor perceived through any of the other senses. Nevertheless, to practitioners of Ayurveda these invisible life forces are very real. They can move, increase or diminish, and they are interrelated as if they were bound together by countless imperceptible threads. Each dosha affects the physical body: the cells, tissues and organs. In addition to its influence on bodily functions, each dosha governs a spiritual and mental activity. The far-reaching functions of the three doshas spring from their individual characteristics.

**Tangible life
energies**

According to Indian philosophy the tridoshas are composed of the five fundamental elements: space, air, fire, water and earth. They are made up in different combinations. Vata is a combination of space and air. Pitta represents fire, with water as a secondary element. Kapha is composed of water and earth.

Principle of the five elements

Characteristics of the three vital forces

Each of the three forces has certain characteristics that are associated with it.

Vata

■ The characteristics of vata reflect those of space and air and are expressed through such words as penetrating, light, mobile, subtle, cold, dry and rough. As an energy force in the body, vata drives all the physical functions that involve movement. It governs the muscles and regulates the internal organs, circulation, breathing and the body's elimination processes. Vata is also responsible for intellectual activity and our sensory organs, and therefore influences mental lucidity, alertness and our ability to learn.

Pitta

■ Pitta, the fiery force, relates to bodily functions that are concerned with heat. It is responsible for regulating body temperature, digestion and metabolism. Pitta also governs blood formation, skin and perception. On the mental and spiritual level, pitta is involved with intellect and emotion. The descriptive qualities of pitta are hot, light, fluid, flowing, acidic, sharp and penetrating.

Kapha

■ Kapha has watery and earthy qualities. Its descriptive words include heavy, cold, soft, sweet, stable, slow and oily. Kapha controls the structure of the body, its stability, flexibility and suppleness. It is responsible for the formation of cells, including the skeleton and the joints. In addition, it governs our resistance to disease. On the spiritual level it regulates mental stability, balance, memory function and compassion.

Total health through balance and harmony

Vitality and
the body's
defences

When all three doshas are fully functional and interacting smoothly, the organism is in equilibrium, and the person is healthy. Ideally, this condition should be constantly maintained: when the doshas are functioning properly this not only reinforces our natural resistance to imbalance and disease, but it also maximises our vitality.

According to Ayurvedic theory, we can achieve this perfect harmony only if we ensure that our potential for physical and spiritual health is constantly developing.

What influences the doshas?

Ayurveda highlights three factors that can unbalance our energy forces of vata, pitta and kapha:

■ If our sensory organs are overtaxed and overstimulated, or conversely if they are understimulated. Traffic noise, air pollution, rushing about, the pressures of time or of too many people around us – all these are part of our everyday experience. We are not always in a position to protect our senses from overstimulation and possible damage. At the opposite end of the scale, we can simply switch off and withdraw – especially if pressure becomes too great – which can be equally damaging to our energy balance.

Pay attention
to the body's
warning
signals

■ If the mind and senses are inappropriately used and the body abused. All too many of us live lifestyles that are too hectic. We are preoccupied with thoughts of performance and material gain, only considering our health if it impedes our ability to function effectively in our everyday lives. Most of us forget that the body is not a machine which needs only an occasional overhaul to keep it in good working order.

According to Ayurvedic theory, a person's susceptibility to certain complaints depends upon their physical and psychological make-up. Ayurveda teaches us to listen to our bodies and to reject a way of life if it puts our health at risk.

■ Time – that is to say the rhythm of day and night, the changing seasons of the year – and age exert an influence. Those who are always working against their internal clock, paying too little attention to life's natural phases of rest and activity, will run the risk, temporarily or permanently, of throwing their energy forces off balance.

Living by our "internal clock"

These are only a few examples of the factors that make our lives difficult. We all have our personal stress patterns, just as we also have our ways of coping – up to point – with life's pressures and with any bad eating habits that can cause imbalance.

The seven stages of imbalance

As soon as we overstep the limits of our ability to cope, our energy forces become unbalanced. When this happens the three doshas can either increase or diminish. They are inhibited, blocked, over- or understimulated. Any one of the three energies – vata, pitta or kapha – can become 'stuck' somewhere in the tissues, or a high concentration of one or other energy can find its way to completely the wrong parts of the body.

According to Ayurveda, such imbalance develops into physical complaints over seven stages:

1 A variety of negative influences cause one or more doshas to build up.

Imbalance of the doshas

2 As long as the disruptive influences are present, the doshas become even more seriously unbalanced. This second stage is known as *aggravation*.

3 The previously localized doshic imbalance spreads to other parts of the body in a process known as *dispersion*.

4 The affected dosha spreads and relocates elsewhere in the body, causing an accumulation of waste products.

5 In the part of the body where the dosha is deposited, the first mild symptoms of sickness begin to appear, which can then

6 develop into acute illness, which may then

7 worsen to become a chronic condition.

Ayurvedic diagnostic techniques aim to spot the early warning signs of doshic imbalance.

Prevention of disease If the first four stages of imbalance are diagnosed and managed by therapeutic procedures, it is often possible to ward off the development of illness or disease.

Ayurveda's main concern is to prevent disease – to stop illnesses breaking out in the first place. When they do occur, Ayurveda promotes healing in the true sense of the word: to make whole. The recovered patient is complete, since his or her life energies are restored to a state of balance and harmony.

Health equals wholeness

Ayurvedic constitutional types

Vata, pitta and kapha are three vital forces which regulate both physical and mental energy. They are present in each of us, but to different degrees and in different combinations which vary from one person to another. According to Ayurvedic belief, the three energies govern our physical and psychological make-up. This means that the predominant forces within each individual define:

- outward physical appearance
- function of the internal organs
- type of intellectual capacity
- individual psychological patterns

Defined by the doshas

Each individual can be categorized as a vata, pitta or kapha type. It is rare for a dosha in its purest form to exist in any one person: most people possess a combination of elements from the doshas. Ayurveda distinguishes between not three but seven constitutional types. In addition to the three pure forms described on the following pages, individuals may be identified as vata-pitta, pitta-kapha, vata-kapha and vata-pitta-kapha.

Constitutional types

Important

The Ayurvedic definition of constitutional types does not divide characteristics into 'good' or 'bad'. Every quality is seen as neutral. Each constitutional type has its strengths and weaknesses. The greatest advantage of recognizing all the positive and negative forces within ourselves is that it makes it possible to diagnose ailments accurately. Ayurveda can reveal in great detail the kind of illnesses to which people of a specific constitutional type may be susceptible, as well as their reaction to diet, climate, season of the year or time of day. The definition of constitutional type can also show how we express our feelings, organize our lives and relate to our environment.

Vata

Vata – main element air

With air as the predominant element, the vata type is likely to react quickly and be sensitive to change. This can mean that the vata type is easily excited and can often feel agitated.

If you are a vata type you could well have a classic 'stress personality' in which pure stimulation can easily spiral into agitation. Your guiding principle should be to try to give yourself plenty of time to relax and live your life at a steady pace.

King of the doshas

Vata disturbance also produces imbalance between pitta and kapha, because vata is the strongest force of the three. As 'king of the doshas' it rules and activates the other two. Vata is the force responsible for movement. Stress-related and psychosomatic ailments are often caused by superfluous vata energy.

Vata characteristics include:

- light weight, thin and tall, slight build
- skin tending to dryness
- irregular appetite and irregular digestion
- tendency towards constipation
- tendency towards flatulence
- light, disturbed sleep
- capacity for great enthusiasm
- ability to learn very quickly but also to forget quickly
- speed of action
- tendency to worry

Signs of vata disturbance

Symptoms of vata imbalance include: rough skin, brittle, rough finger nails, dry tongue and greyish-brown complexion. Because of their tendency to dryness, vata types suffer from constipation and dry stools. Weight loss and "nervous" stomach upsets are also typical vata complaints.

Vata types may also suffer from dizziness, high blood pressure, muscle tension, nerve pain and painful joints, trembling, cramps and shivering.

On the emotional level, vata people are prone to restlessness, sleeplessness, anxiety, worry and depression.

Causes of vata disturbance

The symptoms described above are usually caused by the kind of situations in which vata people often find themselves. Typically, these involve too much activity and too little relaxation. At the same time, overindulgence in rich foods, alcohol or tobacco, sudden or drastic life changes, and too much physical or emotional strain can cause vata imbalance over a long period. Skipping meals, too much cold, raw or dry food, too little sleep, cold, windy weather and excessive travelling can all lead to vata disturbance.

Signs of balanced vata

When vata is undisturbed, people of this constitutional type have a positive and stable prevailing mood. Intellectually and emotionally they are lucid, alert and creative. The ability to act quickly and adapt to different situations are further signs of vata harmony.

Balanced vata
With their predominant dosha in healthy equilibrium, vata types gain the benefits of restful sleep and have efficient excretory functions of both bladder and bowels. Their natural resistance to disease is excellent.

Pitta

Pitta – main element fire

The predominant element of pitta is fire. In general, pitta types enjoy good health. They have good digestion which enables them to build up healthy tissues, so reinforcing their bodies' natural defences. However, some pitta individuals have to learn to strike a balance between activity and relaxation: pitta types can have so much energy that they demand too much of themselves, overstepping their stress limits.

Pitta characteristics include:

- medium build
- normal skin
- tendency to freckles and moles
- large appetite, good digestion
- preference for cold food and drink
- dislike of skipping meals
- aversion to hot weather
- average mental grasp and memory
- average speed of activity
- a way with words, sharp intellect
- quick to anger if excited

Signs of pitta disturbance

Pitta imbalance

Physical symptoms of pitta imbalance include: slightly yellowish complexion, profuse sweating, hot flushes, bad breath, sleep disturbances, poor digestion, inefficient liver function and disturbances of enzymes and hormones. Other signs are inflammation, eczema, bleeding, as well as heartburn, kidney or gallstones, stomach or intestinal ulcers, excessive hunger and thirst, and skin complaints.

On the psychological and emotional level, sufferers from pitta imbalance may become aggressive, hypercritical, stubborn and insensitive.

Causes of pitta disturbance

If you are a pitta type, too much stress, pressure and rushing about can throw your main dosha off balance. It may be because, through lack of time, you skip a meal; or in a crisis situation, you might be unable to express your anger and discontent.

If you belong to the pitta constitutional type you may not be able to tolerate long exposure to heat or sun, or eat food that is too salty, too greasy or too spicy. You may also crave ice cream and cold drinks, and prefer liquids to solid food.

Balancing the "inner fire"

Signs of balanced pitta

If you are a pitta type and your fiery element is well balanced, you will experience inner peace and contentment. This pleasant, satisfying feeling fills you with energy and encourages you to be adventurous. In a balanced state your digestion is excellent, your body graceful and supple. If your 'inner fire' is in equilibrium you will not experience problems with either hot flushes or inflammation that can often trouble pitta types.

Kapha

Kapha – main elements earth and water

People governed by the water-earth element are calm, settled and stable. The governing kapha dosha is not easily disturbed, so the general health of kapha types is usually good. Nevertheless, kapha types must pay attention to their well-being, especially as their slow life rhythm can cause them to sink into boredom, lack of ambition and physical inertia.

Lack of stimulation can lead to negative stress – in other words to imbalance – in this constitutional type. For this reason kapha personalities should aim to strike a balance between active and passive behaviour.

Kapha characteristics include:

- solid, heavy build
- tendency to smooth, oily skin
- abundant, usually dark hair
- small appetite, slow digestion
- regular bowel movements
- long, deep sleep
- aversion to foggy weather
- slow to learn but good memory
- slow, methodical activity
- slow arousal and excitability
- calm, stable personality
- pleasant, "happy-go-lucky" attitude

Signs of kapha disturbance

Difficult though it is to unbalance kapha energy, if it does become disturbed the following symptoms occur: pale skin and extreme sensitivity to cold. A feeling of heaviness, especially first thing in the morning, is a typical sign of a kapha imbalance. Kapha types are also inclined to put on weight, to sleep too much and too long, and to slow down their whole rhythm of life.

Kapha
imbalance

Physical disturbances include problems with the respiratory tract, such as excess mucus, colds, bronchitis and blocked sinuses, as well as fluid retention and heaviness in the limbs. Kapha types are also prone to allergies and diabetes. On the emotional and psychological level, a kapha imbalance will cause kapha types to put off jobs they really ought to do and to avoid change. Their vitality and receptivity are drastically reduced and they often suffer from depression.

Causes of kapha disturbance

As we have already said, a lack of stimulation and not having enough to do are major causes of kapha imbalance. Other reasons include overeating, or eating a diet which includes too much sugar, fat or salt. Insufficient exercise, too much sleep, and cold, damp weather can also throw the kapha constitutional type off balance for long periods.

Imbalance of the water– earth element

Signs of kapha balance

Kapha types whose water–earth element is in equilibrium are physically strong, with well-knit joints and well-proportioned bodies. They glow with inner calm and are compassionate, patient, courageous, vigorous and mentally stable.

Important

You may recognize yourself in one or other of these broad descriptions of the constitutional types. People often identify readily with the Ayurvedic categories. However, the selection of factors listed here represent only a few of the many aspects that go to make up a human being. They are in no way a reflection of the whole range of personal characteristics. Only a qualified, experienced Ayurvedic practitioner can carry out a complete analysis of your constitutional type with all its strengths and weaknesses.

What can Ayurveda achieve for you?

Ayurveda is a holistic system of healing concerned with every aspect of human life: mind, body, behaviour and environment. The primary focus of Ayurveda is on preventing illness in the first place, and then on treating illness when it does occur. It also seeks to improve our own spiritual, intellectual and physical ability to heal ourselves.

Holistic prevention and cure

According to theories formulated by Indian healers thousands of years ago, if we adopt a healthy lifestyle suited to our own constitutional type, we shall succeed in achieving and maintaining our well-being. However, we have to take responsibility for our health. Our life's ambition and effort should be to raise our own awareness and discover who we really are. Inherent in this is to observe the laws of nature and follow a healthy diet.

If, despite taking these preventive measures, our inner equilibrium is still disturbed, Ayurveda is able to heal. Ayurvedic theory is applied in two areas:

1 Guided by Ayurvedic teachings you can learn to recognize and treat doshic imbalances caused by diet or stress. You can also learn how to avoid such imbalances in the future.

2 If you are in good general health, Ayurveda can help you to adjust your lifestyle so that you will feel noticeably more contented and balanced than ever before. It can teach you how to apply your mental and physical powers to the full, and help you develop a level of calm detachment that will enable you to face up to the stresses of everyday life. Through a process of 'inner purification', you can achieve a marked increase in your energy levels and learn to pay greater attention to your own needs, so bringing yourself into harmony with your inner nature. You will feel both physically and emotionally more dynamic and balanced, and so feel a greater zest for life.

Inner purification

Self-help with Ayurveda

Not all Ayurvedic practices are suitable as self-help methods; some require extensive understanding of Ayurvedic concepts and the supervision of a trained therapist. In this book, we only recommend self-help methods that you can safely carry out by yourself. You should consider the following points:

■ The theories discussed here go to make up a philosophy of life. They are not simply a matter of abstract ideas, they involve practical applications and exercises.

Exercises for every day

   Instinctively, you may have already put some Ayurvedic theories into practice in your own life. However, what one person may take for granted might mean a complete change of deep-rooted habits for another. Ayurveda can only make a real impact if it becomes part of your everyday way of life.

   Ayurveda will have little effect on your overall well-being if all you do is meditate now and again, or do the occasional yoga or breathing exercise, while otherwise carrying on in the same old unhealthy way. Ayurveda demands more than this if you want to become physically, mentally and emotionally fit in the Ayurvedic sense, and then stay that way in the long term. Its teachings do not provide a quick-fix programme leading to dramatic health improvements in the shortest possible time. In order to achieve long-term success and genuine results with Ayurveda, you must persevere over a long period and incorporate Ayurvedic principles into your daily life.

Practice makes perfect

Regular practice

If you follow Ayurvedic health guidelines, regularly perform the exercises, and live according to the teachings of Ayurveda, you will learn how to recognize and avoid many of the physical and emotional problems that crop up from day to day.

● The questionnaire (see pages 29-31) will help you assess your constitutional type. This knowledge will not only enhance your self-awareness, it will also help you to have more faith in the wisdom of your own body and to avoid negative influences.

Boosting our self-healing powers

- You will help your body to recover more quickly the equilibrium it loses through a whole series of disruptive factors.
- Inner purification not only rids your body of harmful waste products and toxins, it can also help to eliminate the mental and emotional baggage that can lead to illness, and boost your physical and psychological self-healing powers.

Ayurvedic therapy

If you seek treatment from a trained Ayurvedic practitioner, you will first undergo a thorough diagnostic examination. One of the most important stages of this examination is the pulse diagnosis. Unlike in conventional Western medicine, in which a doctor takes your pulse to check your heart rate, an Ayurvedic practitioner uses the pulse to ascertain the state of your doshas, or energies, and what is happening throughout your body. By asking questions and observing external signs – the skin, hair, finger nails, eyes – the therapist can determine your constitutional type and design a suitable programme of therapy.

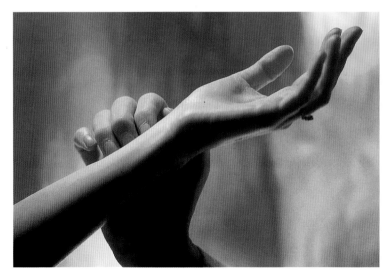

Pulse diagnosis

The fundamental Ayurvedic therapy is *Panchakarma*, a purification procedure designed to rid the body of metabolic waste, environmental pollution and undigested food. Ayurveda calls this waste product *ama*, which means "unripe" or "undigested". Obstructions caused by ama in the body are regarded as one of the main causes of illness, general malaise and inefficient performance.

Ayurveda – a far-reaching form of therapy

Ama can also accumulate on the psychological level as a result of feelings that remain "undigested" – in other words, that have not been worked through properly. Likewise, unresolved conflicts and stressful experiences can cause problems. As part of a Panchakarma programme, you may be prescribed a purification diet. You may also undergo various forms of massage, that are both relaxing and enjoyable. One of the most pleasant and restful treatment experiences is a combination of *Shirodhara*, in which warm – not hot – Shirodhara (sesame oil) is trickled over the forehead, and *Abhyanga*, or "loving hands" massage, are carried out simultaneously.

It is always important to remember during the course of an Ayurvedic cure that it takes more than a physical overhaul to achieve good health. A supervised Ayurvedic treatment may involve instruction in additional forms of therapy and relaxation techniques, such as breathing, yoga exercises, and meditation.

The way to perfect health

■ Ayurveda is a holistic system of healing. All techniques are aimed at achieving not just physical but also mental and spiritual harmony, since many diseases originate in negative thinking.

Important

While Ayurvedic methods can easily be applied to all areas of life and to all individuals, they must be practised carefully and thoughtfully. You should not attempt to use Ayurvedic methods to treat yourself for chronic illness or serious acute conditions without first consulting your family doctor and a trained Ayurvedic practitioner. If in doubt, SEEK MEDICAL ADVICE. Ayurvedic exercises can always be used to supplement medically prescribed treatment at home.

How Ayurveda can heal

Successful Ayurvedic treatment

Ayurvedic healers claim their therapies are successful in treating many conditions, in particular those in which orthodox medicine can only deal with the symptoms. This applies above all to chronic complaints of the neurovegetative system, in which the part played by mental and emotional factors cannot be underestimated. Ayurveda has been found to be effective in the treatment of:

● Irregularity of autonomic bodily functions: sleep disturbances, tension headaches, migraine, neurovegetative dystonia, depression, anxiety states, heart conditions of nervous origin, such as rapid or irregular pulse, and palpitations.
● Gynaecological problems: menstrual and menopausal difficulties, over- and underweight.
● Coronary and circulatory problems: high blood pressure, angina, rapid or irregular pulse, and palpitations.
● Digestive disorders: underactive bowels and chronic digestive problems, such as flatulence, constipation, acid indigestion and heartburn; chronic gastritis, stomach ulcers, haemorrhoids.
● Metabolic disorders: excess cholesterol and uric acid, diabetes, rheumatism.
● Degenerative conditions of the joints and spinal column: chronic pain, muscle tension, and conditions impeding movement, such as stiff joints; sciatica.
● Chronic inflammation: sinus trouble, chronic bronchitis.
● Allergic conditions: bronchial asthma, hay fever.
● Skin complaints: acne, psoriasis, dermatitis, eczema.
● Problems of old age: osteoporosis, memory failings.

Techniques to aid recovery

Ayurvedic therapy can also provide support for those who wish to give up alcohol, smoking or prescribed drugs. It also offers aftercare techniques to aid recuperation after major operations or long-term illness.

Self-analysis: discover your constitutional type

Each individual is unique. In this sense, it is not only impossible to pigeon-hole people, it is also somewhat pointless. However, classification according to type can be useful and is possible in certain areas, such as body shape and build, personal likes and dislikes, and behaviour patterns. Ayurveda uses such categories as a source of information when looking for signs of doshic imbalance.

Discovering who you are

The main purpose of the questionnaire on pages 29 to 31 is to encourage you to reflect calmly about yourself and thus help you come a little closer to knowing who you are. In the modern world, it is becoming increasingly obvious that many of us have lost touch with our real selves. We neither recognize our personal strengths and weaknesses, nor do we have much idea of what is good for us and what is not.

Before studying the exercises, you are advised first to complete the questionnaire. The answers you get should help you to:

Recognizing your strengths and weaknesses

- understand, according to your constitutional type, the steps you should take to stay healthy;
- know what treatment to adopt if you are ill;
- understand yourself better, for example why you dislike certain foods, why you overreact in certain situations, or why you sometimes feel over-tired and depressed.

Important

This personal analysis is not a substitute for a thorough medical examination and type classification. Trained Ayurvedic practitioners follow a different procedure.

Introduction

The following self-analysis test consists of 60 statements, divided into three sections covering the vata, pitta and kapha energies. Think about each statement carefully and consider to what extent it applies to you, then mark your response with a tick on the scale of 0 to 6. If you have difficulty answering some questions, let yourself be guided by how you have usually felt throughout your

Your temperament? life – or at least over the past few years. Consider your prevailing mood or your predominant attitude to life. This applies particularly to questions involving mental and emotional characteristics.

Evaluation

When you have filled in each section of the questionnaire, add up the ticks. First add up your score for the VATA test, then do the same for the PITTA and KAPHA questionnaires. Now compare your three scores: you will see whether one type outweighs the others, or whether perhaps two types predominate, or even if all three apply more or less equally. You can then judge which type you are: For example:

Pitta 80, Vata 61 (Kapha 29)	=	Pitta-Vata type
Vata 88, (Pitta 34, Kapha 37)	=	Vata type
Vata 61, Pitta 64, Kapha 60	=	Vata-Pitta-Kapha type

On pages 15 to 21 you will find brief descriptions of the main physical, mental and emotional features of the three types. The dosha for which you have the highest score is the one that has the greatest influence on you at present. As you consider the practical exercises, you should concentrate mainly on that dosha. If you are a mixed constitutional type, read the instructions for **Let your** both types. Be guided by your feelings in deciding to what extent **feelings** each statement applies to you and which exercises will benefit you **guide you** most at a given time.

Discover your constitutional type

Vata Test

	never/rarely		sometimes			usually	
	0	1	2	3	4	5	6

1. I act quickly.
2. I find it hard to learn and to remember things for long.
3. I am lively and enthusiastic.
4. I am of light build and have difficulty gaining weight.
5. I am receptive to new ideas.
6. I walk quickly and lightly.
7. I find it hard to make decisions.
8. I am prone to flatulence or constipation.
9. I often have cold hands and feet.
10. I am often worried and anxious.
11. I tolerate cold weather less well than other people.
12. I speak quickly and my friends find me very talkative.
13. My moods change quickly and I react according to how I am feeling.
14. I often sleep badly and often wake up in the night.
15. My skin tends to be dry, especially in winter.
16. I have a very active mind, bubbling over with ideas, and occasionally restless.
17. My movements are swift and vigorous, and I have sudden bursts of energy.
18. I am easily excited.
19. Left to my own devices, I have irregular eating and sleeping habits.
20. I am sensitive to draughts.

Total Vata Score:

Pitta Test

	never/rarely 0 1	sometimes 2 3 4	usually 5 6

1. I consider myself very efficient.
2. Everything I do is precise and deliberate.
3. I am strong willed and can usually get my own way.
4. In hot, humid weather, I feel unwell and tire easily.
5. I sweat easily.
6. Although I don't always show it, I am often irritated or angry.
7. I am uneasy if I have to miss a meal or eat later than usual.
8. My hair has at least one of the following characteristics: prematurely grey or balding; thin, silky, smooth; red or with reddish tints.
9. I have a good appetite and can eat large quantities.
10. Many people consider me obstinate.
11. I have a regular digestion; I am more prone to diarrhoea than constipation.
12. I easily lose patience.
13. I am inclined to be a perfectionist.
14. I quickly lose my temper, but forget just as quickly.
15. I like cold food and chilled drinks.
16. I am very direct and rather an extrovert.
17. I cannot tolerate highly seasoned or hot food.
18. I am not as tolerant as I should be.
19. I enjoy challenges and I am very tenacious in achieving my goal.
20. I am highly critical of myself and others.

Total Pitta Score:

Kapha Test

	never/rarely		sometimes			usually	
	0	1	2	3	4	5	6

1. I usually act slowly and unhurriedly.
2. I gain weight more quickly and find it harder to lose weight than other people.
3. I am very calm and placid by nature and rarely lose my self-control.
4. I do not mind missing meals.
5. I am prone to excess mucus/catarrh, chronic constipation or asthma.
6. I need at least eight hours' sleep if I am to feel good the following day.
7. I sleep soundly.
8. I seldom become angry.
9. I learn more slowly than others, but have an excellent long-term memory.
10. I do not have problems handling money.
11. I detest cold, damp weather.
12. My hair is abundant, dark and wavy or coarse.
13. I have soft, smooth, pale skin.
14. I am heavily built.
15. By nature I am cheerful, gentle, loving and very forgiving.
16. My digestion is regular, even when travelling.
17. I have good staying power and resistance, my energy level is constant.
18. I walk at a slow and measured pace.
19. I tend to oversleep and it takes me time to wake up in the morning.
20. I eat slowly, methodically and with attention.

Total Kapha Score:

From: Gottwald/Howald: *Ayurveda im Business*. mvg – Moderne Verlagsgesellschaft GmbH, Munich; 1992.

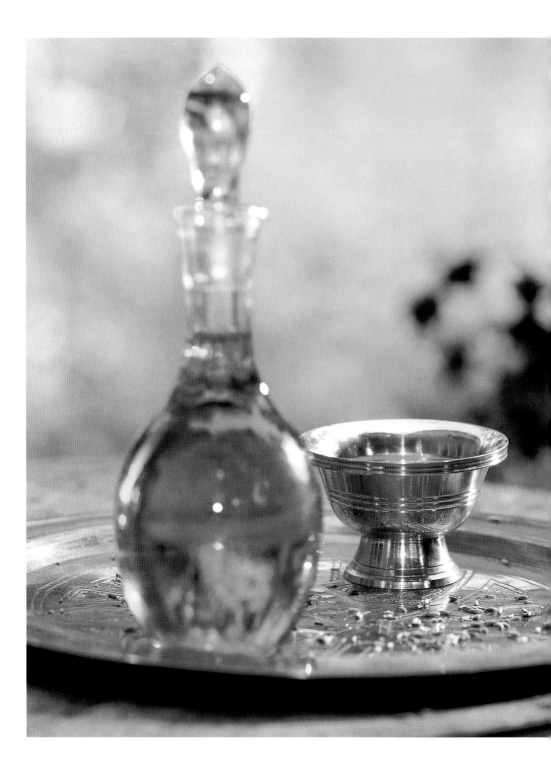

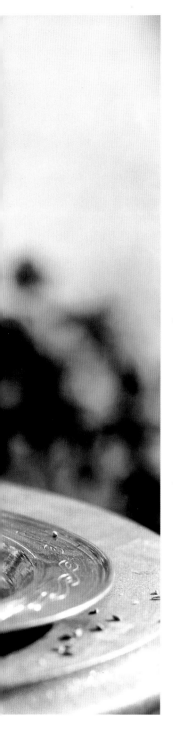

Health lies within ourselves

"The Ayurvedic expression for health is swastha, *which means 'to be rooted in oneself'. From the vedic point of view, the self is our deepest inner level of being, a place of tranquil consciousness where each of us is in touch with and at one with the entire cosmos. It is the level of human existence which gives the healthy individual a feeling of identity and inner wholeness."*
Dr Ernst Schrott

These days, many people have lost contact with their true selves. According to Ayurvedic belief the lack of this knowledge – the loss of the natural wisdom of body and soul – is the origin of sickness and suffering. The exercises on the following pages can help you learn once again to pay heed to your true self.

The Ayurvedic approach to health and healing

According to ancient vedic tradition, there exists within each human a place of perfect well-being. This sacred place is situated at the deepest level of our consciousness and only when we are completely at peace can we find the inner path that leads there.

The holistic system of Ayurveda shows us the way to reach that serene, tranquil place. In recovering the natural equilibrium between your vital energies, you will take a great and crucial step towards reaching your optimum health.

In Ayurvedic terms, health means harmony between the three doshas – the driving forces of vata, pitta and kapha. The focal point of the Ayurvedic approach is to achieve balance between the three doshas.

The next few pages will introduce you to a number of therapeutic possibilities. The exercises, which you can easily do at home, have been divided into two sections which represent two stages of an Ayurvedic cure. These are

Health means balanced energies

known as *purification* (see below) and *regeneration* (see page 42). A whole chapter is devoted to the third stage, *diet* (page 71). There you will find valuable advice about healthy eating, as well as particular recommendations for a diet to suit your constitutional type.

Purification

Before beginning the programme of exercises, you must rid your body of ama – toxins and waste products. The 10-day diet cure opposite aims specifically to eliminate toxins and waste products from the body.

Usually, purification therapy consists of a light diet, which has the added benefit of improving your digestion. Whether you are taking supervised treatment with a practitioner, or trying out a self-help programme at home, it is recommended that you make the purification process of cleansing the body your first step.

Cleansing the body

Ama therapy at home

Follow this diet for 10 days:

Your purification diet

● **Morning:** On rising, drink a glass of warm, boiled water with a teaspoon of freshly squeezed lemon juice and one or two teaspoons of good-quality honey. The water should not be too hot, otherwise the honey loses much of its goodness. You can skip breakfast, but if you feel very hungry drink some freshly squeezed fruit juice or eat a little toast.

● **Lunch:** At midday you should take a light, warm meal, eating enough to satisfy your hunger. Pay close attention to your personal "saturation point", in order to avoid overeating. Try to eat in a peaceful atmosphere, and sit quietly for 10 minutes after your meal.

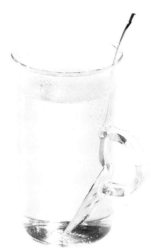

Hot water

● **Dinner:** You can miss dinner. If you feel very hungry, however, you may drink fruit juice as at breakfast time or soup made with cereal, rice or vegetables. You can also eat rice and vegetables. In any case, the evening meal must be eaten between six and seven o'clock.

● **Between meals:** You should not eat between the main meals, but if you are very hungry, fruit juice is allowed.

● **Hot water:** This is the most important component of an Ayurveda cure: it stimulates the metabolism and encourages the elimination of ama. Drink the hot water in small sips and drink just enough to quench your thirst – half a cup each

Drink hot water

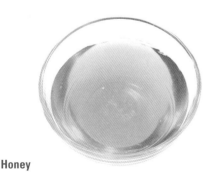

Honey

Enough to quench your thirst

time is usually enough. Boil the water for at least 10 minutes. This improves the taste and also helps it to penetrate the body's cells more easily. Keep it in a thermos flask, so that it stays at the right temperature to drink.

▶ Avoid the following during the cure: roast, fried, fatty or sour foods; uncooked foods, including raw vegetables and raw-grain muesli; fish, pork and beef; cheese, quark and curd cheese; yoghurt and other sour milk products; sweet foods.

▶ The following foods are recommended during the cure: basmati rice; cooked leaf vegetables, carrots, and

beetroot; mung beans; bread produced by natural proving methods, using organically produced flour; small quantities of fresh salad; soups made with vegetables or grains.

Important

After 10 days, gradually start to eat normally. Be guided by the chapter "Eating what the body needs" (see page 71). In addition, you are advised to continue drinking boiled, hot water every one or two hours.

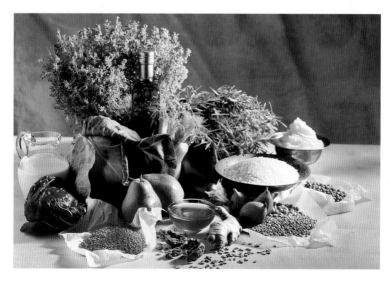

Some of the foods you should eat during the 10-day purification cure

Top-to-toe massage

Ayurvedic practitioners
recommend regular massage as
a technique to encourage the
release of toxins and waste
products from the body.
Massaging the skin stimulates
blood circulation and
encourages the flow of lymph,
so speeding up the elimination
of ama. Vegetable oil massaged
into the skin also provides the
body with valuable
nourishment. At the same time,
massage is a soothing and
stabilizing process that benefits
body, mind and spirit.

Regular massage For all of these reasons,
massage is part of the
purification therapy known as
Panchakarma (see page 25),
supplementing the diet cure.
For home use, Ayurveda
recommends that self-massage
should be carried out as part of
your normal morning routine.

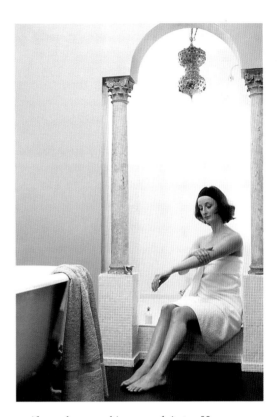

Oil Massage

Vata types should include a
daily oil massage in their
programme, while kapha and
pitta types should do so only
two or three times a week. The
recommended lubricant and
embrocation is high-quality,
cold-pressed sesame oil.
If you are a pitta type, however,

or if you have a skin complaint,
you should use olive, coconut
or sweet almond oil instead.
All these oils are available
from pharmacists and health
food shops.

Massage gently with oil

Whatever oil you use, before
you use it for the first time,
you must prepare it as follows:
● Heat the oil gently in a
saucepan to about 110°C. To
check the temperature, either
use a thermometer or drip a
couple of drops of water into

The Ayurvedic approach to health and healing

Preparing the oil

the hot oil: if the temperature is right, you will hear a sizzling sound as the water hits the oil. The oil is now "ripe" and thus more suitable for massage. It will also keep longer. Prepare the oil in quantities of 100 to 200 ml, and store it in a glass bottle.

Important

Allow hot oil to cool to body temperature before using it for massage.

Before each massage, pour as much oil as you need into a small bowl. Stand the bowl over a pan of boiling water until it reaches body temperature (37°C/98.4°F).

Warm oil is not only more pleasant to use, it also penetrates the skin more easily.

▶ Massage yourself before your bath or shower:

● Sit on a low stool or on the floor, on a bath mat or towel.

● Apply the warm oil all over your body from head to foot. The skin should absorb the oil before you begin the massage.

● To help your skin absorb the oil, use up-and-down or circular movements of your hands, repeating each movement at least three times as you smooth the oil into your skin.

Oil massage in the morning

Massage your forehead with your fingertips

Head • When you have oiled your whole body, start slowly to massage your scalp. Place your fingertips on your head and massage as though you were . washing your hair. Massage slowly and carefully, starting at the hairline and working backwards over the sides of your head to your neck.

Ears • Next, massage both your ears simultaneously. Hold your earlobes between thumb and forefinger and gently move your thumbs up and down.

Forehead • Then place your fingertips in the centre of your forehead. Using gentle pressure, move your fingers outwards towards the temples, then massage the temples with a circular movement.

Chin • When you have massaged your temples, move your fingertips down your cheeks to your chin. Use the same horizontal strokes on your chin as you did on your forehead, Then place your two index fingers on either side of your nose and massage gently up and down.

Neck and throat • Now we come to the neck and throat. Lay one hand on each shoulder blade, and

massage up and down towards the roots of your hair. Use only gentle stroking movements on your throat – working with one hand at a time – starting at the level of your collar bones and working upwards towards the chin.

• Press down firmly as you massage your arms, and use circular movements for the joints. Massage first your right arm, then your left, stroking up and down. Massage the shoulder joints with small spiral movements, and your upper arms with up-and-down strokes. Use circular movements to massage your elbows and armpits, then do the same on your knuckles. Hold each finger individually and stroke it gently towards the nail. **Press down firmly**

• Massage your chest with gentle, circular movements, women should massage around the breasts. Use gentle up-and-down strokes along the breastbone. Then lay your right hand flat on your abdomen, letting your left hand rest by your side. **Massage gently**

• Massage your abdomen with your right hand using circular, clockwise movements. Start with small circles, then **Gentle circular movements** increase gradually until you are massaging your whole abdomen with large, circular movements. Rest your right hand and repeat the process with your left hand.

● Now massage your back and buttocks. You will only be able to reach your lower back when massaging yourself. Stand up and lay the palms of **Massage** your hands on your lower back **vigorously** and massage vigorously up and down, then massage your buttocks, using the same, vigorous movement.

● Sit down again to massage your legs. Use the same procedure as for the arms. Massage first the right leg then the left. Use circular movements to massage your knee and ankle joints. To massage your calf and thigh muscles, use up-and-down strokes, pressing firmly.

● Finally, the foot massage. **Massage the** You should take extra care in **reflex points** massaging your feet, as they **in your feet** contain many important reflex points. Massage first your right foot, then your left.

● Place one hand over the instep and the other one on the sole. Stroke gently, starting at the tips of the toes and working upwards towards the ankle, then slide your hands back to the toes.

● Now lay your thumbs side by side on the underside of your heel. Massage firmly with your thumbs, using small spiral movements, working along the sole towards the toes. When you reach the toes, slide your thumbs down your foot again, pressing down firmly.

● Next, the toes. Support your **Massage** foot with one hand and gently **each toe** stroke one toe at a time, working from the joint to the tip. Then gently pull each toe. Now massage between your toes. Supporting the foot with one hand, take the skin between the toes between the thumb and forefinger of the other hand. Squeeze the skin gently then pull it firmly forward, towards the tips of the toes.

Important

Women should avoid oil massage during the first three days of a period. If your skin is sensitive and the sesame oil makes it itch – though this is rare – you must use olive, coconut or almond oil.

You should spend about 10 minutes on your massage, and then relax for another five minutes to allow your skin to absorb the oil.

Take your time After oil massage, Ayurveda recommends a warm bath or shower. The water should not be too hot and you should use mild soap. This leaves a thin film of oil on the skin, which balances vata and keeps the muscles warm.

Dry massage

More potent A more intense massage technique than oil massage is dry massage using raw silk gloves. You can buy these gloves in pharmacies and medical suppliers, although you may have to order them specially.

Dry massage is highly stimulating for connective tissues, circulation and metabolism and is specially beneficial if you have greasy skin, are overweight or have a slow metabolism.

Kapha types should perform dry massage more frequently than oil massage. Whatever your constitutional type, this is the best form of massage if you feel your body needs

revitalizing – perhaps during a springtime purification cure, or while recovering from an illness, or after a course of prescribed medicines such as antibiotics.

Dry massage in the morning, ● Follow the same procedure and techniques as for oil massage (page 38-40), but spend only about four minutes on a dry massage, immediately after rising in the morning.

Afterwards, Ayurveda recommends a 10-minute soak in a warm bath, to encourage the outflow of waste products and toxins.

Important

Because the circulation is so strongly stimulated by dry massage, people with circulatory disorders should proceed with caution. Even if you do not have such problems, you should not overdo it at the beginning. During the first two weeks you should only massage each part of the body with up-and-down strokes. You can then increase the number of strokes from 10 to 20, and later to 30 then 40.

Regeneration

After the purification ritual has cleaned out and tuned up your body, the following set of exercises will intensify the healing process. In Ayurvedic terms, *regeneration* means restoring and stabilizing the balance of the doshas.

Find the place of inner peace

If you practice Ayurveda over a long period of time, you will become aware that you are getting ever closer to discovering inner peace. You will feel more balanced, more contented than ever before, and will manage to avoid many of the stressful situations that normally exhaust you or even make you ill.

Healthy movement

Movement, in the form of natural activities or specific physical exercise, is very important in Ayurveda.

Physical exercise in Ayurveda, however, does not mean strenuous training routines that make you perspire, or competitive sports for which you have to summon up all your energy reserves. The idea is to enjoy pleasant exercise that, without imposing strain on the body, leaves you feeling revitalized.

Easy and enjoyable exercise

Ayurvedic exercises strive towards an ideal balance and harmony between body and mind. Walking in the countryside comes very close to this ideal, since it is a natural activity which brings all the doshas into equilibrium.

Exercise can, of course, take the form of sport, but in Ayurvedic belief not every kind of sport is equally beneficial to every constitutional type. Refer to the table on page 43 to determine the sport or sports that are best for you.

Find the best activity for you

Tridosha exercises

Ayurveda advises certain types of movement, known as tridosha exercises, to achieve balance between vata, pitta and kapha. The following section (pages 44-56) illustrates and explains three tridosha routines which are basic to Ayurveda:

Movement to bring harmony

● Salute to the Sun – a yogic exercise sequence involving stretching, turning and balance

● A sequence of easy yoga exercises for body and spirit

● Simple yogic breathing exercises – *Pranayama*

Vata	Pitta	Kapha	
Yoga	Skiing	Weightlifting	**The choice**
Dancing	Brisk walking	Tennis	**is yours**
(e.g. Ballet)	or Jogging	Football	
Aerobics	Sailing	Running	
Walking	Horse riding	Dancing	
Hiking (short	Hiking	Aerobics	
distances)	Mountaineering	Rowing	
Cycling	Swimming	Fencing	

Morning exercise ▶ The best time to exercise is in the morning, after you have taken a shower or bath and before breakfast. Set aside about half an hour, so that you can do the exercises without distractions.

Important

Exercise with care: bear in mind how much time you have and how supple you are. Give yourself plenty of time – two or three minutes – for each sequence. With practice, when you are able to adopt the poses without difficulty, you can complete the exercises more quickly. The step-by-step progression avoids the risk of strain or pulled muscles that can occur if you take little daily exercise or do not regularly take part in sport.

Salute to the Sun

This exercise consists of a sequence of 12 postures linked together and flowing smoothly into one another.

The effect is both profound and far-reaching. The various postures, involving either lifting of the limbs or stretching of the muscles, release muscle tension and make the joints more flexible.

In addition, the various sequences of movement have the effect of massaging the internal organs and stimulating circulation.

Relaxing movements

● Back pain, stiff joints or circulatory problems will gradually disappear with the help of these exercises.
If you do them regularly, you will also observe how your spirit is in tune with the sequence of movements performed by your body. You will feel a beneficial harmony between the two. Rhythmic breathing will help you to appreciate the way the exercises flow.

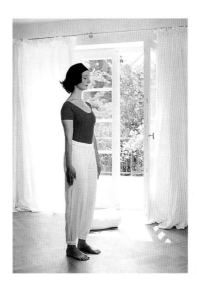

The Mountain

1 The Mountain: Stand erect with your knees relaxed and slightly bent, and your feet side by side (see photograph). Now put the palms of your hands together in front of your chest, then bend your arms and press your breastbone gently with your thumbs.

● In this posture you gather strength and increase your concentration. Take a few seconds to experience these sensations, breathing calmly in and out.

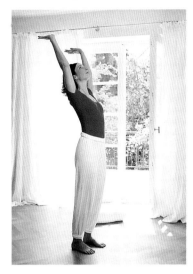

Upward stretch

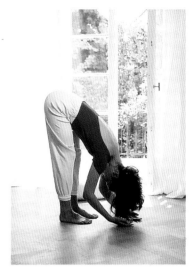

Forward bend

2 Upward stretch: Breath in and out through your nose and slowly raise your arms above your head. Bend your head back and look up to the ceiling. Continue to breathe evenly.

● Take care only to lean back as far as is comfortable for you. Relax in this posture for a few seconds, staying conscious of your body.

3 Forward bend: Breathing out through your mouth, slowly return to the upright position then bend forward as far as possible, until your arms and head are hanging loosely downwards.

● Your back should be straight and your knees slightly bent.
● Breathe normally and think how, with practice, you will become increasingly supple.
● When you have done this exercise often enough, you will be able to lay the palms of your hands flat on the floor, or grasp your feet and touch one knee with your head.

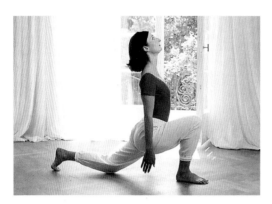
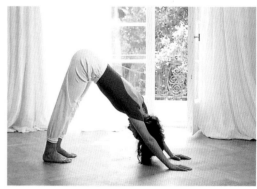

Left leg back

4 Left leg back: As you breathe in, bend your legs, then stretch your left leg out behind you, with your left knee touching the floor. Bend your right leg to provide support.

● Support yourself with the palms of your hands.
● Straighten your back and look up towards the ceiling.
● When you feel more confident with this posture, lift your left knee slightly so that only the tips of your toes and the palms of your hands are touching the floor.
● Don't forget about breathing: breathe calmly, in and out.

5 The Dog – face down: As you breathe out, stretch your right leg behind you so that it is parallel with the left. Supporting yourself with the palms of your hand, lift your hips, keeping your heels touching the floor, and stretching the backs of your legs. Your head should hang loosely between your arms.

● Breathe calmly and evenly while in this posture.
● Remain in this position for a few seconds and feel the sensations in your body.

The Dog – face down

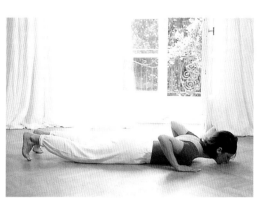
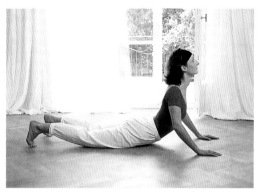

Drop to the floor

6 Drop to the floor: As you breathe out, slowly straighten your body. First let your knees touch the floor, then lower your body until your chest and chin are touching the floor.

● Eight parts of your body should now be touching the floor – both sets of toes, both knees, chest, both hands and your chin.
● You may find this posture very strenuous at the beginning, but it will soon become much easier with practice.
● Make sure you continue to breathe evenly during this exercise.

7 The Cobra – face up: Breathing out, lower your pelvis to the floor and push up with your arms to lift your upper body.

● As you slowly straighten up, bend your neck backwards.
● Breathe calmly and evenly, in and out.
● The stretching of your thorax deepens your breathing – be very conscious of this.

The Cobra– face up

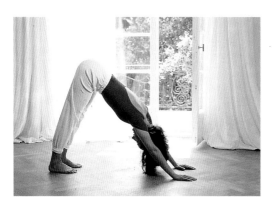

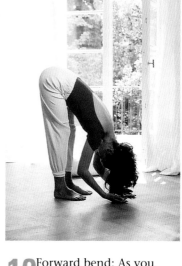

**The Dog –
face down**

8 The Dog – face down:
Breathing out, lift your hips,
returning to the posture
described in position 5.

**Forward
bend**

10 Forward bend: As you
breathe out, bring your
right leg forward and slowly lift
your hips upwards.

● Both legs should now be
stretched, your spine straight
and your head hanging loosely
between your arms.
● This is the same as position 3.

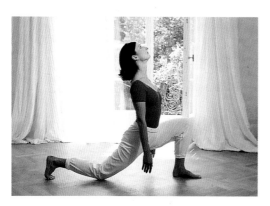

**Right leg
back**

9 Right leg back: As you
breathe out, repeat
position 4, but this time bend
your left leg forward and
stretch your right leg back, with
the knee touching the floor.

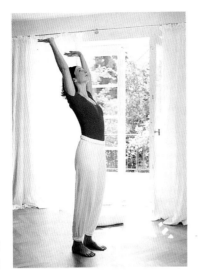

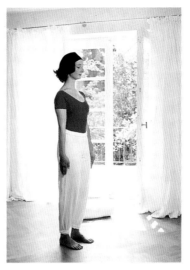

Upward stretch

The Mountain

11 Upward stretch: Now repeat position 2. As you breathe in, lift both arms upwards.

● The stretching movement should stem from the upper back and pelvis, not from the head or neck.
● Look upwards and breathe calmly and evenly.

12 The Mountain: This is the same as position 1.

● As you breathe out, slowly return your upper body to the upright position, moving from the pelvis and upper body – do not start by bringing your head forward!
● Breathe slowly and evenly.
● Look straight ahead, and enjoy the feeling of revitalization.

This posture completes the Salute to the Sun cycle. The sequence can be repeated two to six times. Before each repeated sequence, stand still and take a few breaths.

Yoga exercises for body and spirit

The following selection of yoga exercises are among the basic forms of Ayurvedic therapy. These *asanas*, or postures, are exercises involving stretching, bending, turning and, finally, relaxation.

Each posture has a specific therapeutic effect and benefit. Asanas performed in the sitting position encourage correct alignment of the spinal column and good posture. Bending and turning exercises stimulate digestion and increase the flexibility of the spinal column. The relaxation and breathing exercises are designed to increase alertness and to let the previous exercises take effect.

The best time to carry out this series of exercises is either in the morning or the late afternoon. Each sequence should take between 10 and 15 minutes.

Important

Always perform the exercises slowly and thoughtfully. Never strain yourself. The more you practise, the easier the postures will become. Correct, regular breathing will facilitate movement – never hold your breath or take shallow breaths while doing yoga exercises. As soon as you feel you have had enough, or you find a posture too difficult, stop exercising and relax in the corpse position.

Head-to-knee pose (one minute)

● Sit on the floor and stretch both legs in front of you. Flex your feet so that your toes point towards your head, thus stretching the backs of your legs and your heels.
● Women should now bend their right leg, men the left. Draw up your foot (right foot for women, left foot for men) so that the sole touches the inner thigh of your outstretched leg.
● Breathing in, stretch your arms above your head. As you breathe out, bend your body

Head-to-knee pose

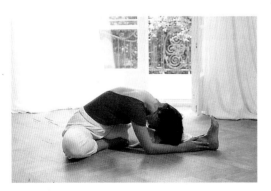

over the outstretched leg, until your forehead touches the knee.

● See photograph page 50 – keep your back straight and do not hunch your shoulders. If you have difficulties, bend the outstretched knee a little, which will relieve the tension in your lower back.

● Hold the position for a few breaths, then straighten up as you breathe in.

● Change legs and perform the exercise on the other side.

Plough pose
(Fifteen seconds to one minute)

● Lie in the corpse position with your arms resting by your sides (1). See photograph below.

● Keeping your legs stretched, bring them up and over your head until the tips of your toes are touching the floor (2). See photograph above. Push your legs as far back as possible so that your chin is touching your chest.

● Fold your arms behind your head (3) or let them rest on the floor alongside your body. Stay in this position for up to one minute, breathing slowly in and out.

● To bring yourself out of the plough pose, support the base of your spine with both hands. As you breathe out, bend your knees and slowly uncurl, one vertebra at a time, until your back is once again flat on the

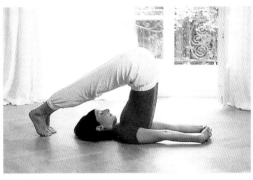

Plough pose (2)

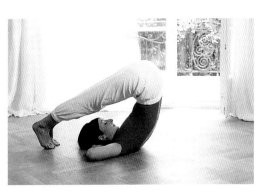

Plough pose (3)

Plough pose (1) – Corpse position

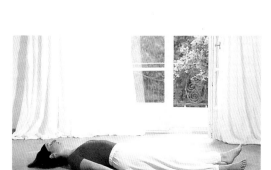

floor, with your legs bent at the knees, and your feet and head on the floor.

● Relax in this position for a few moments.

Cobra pose
(Thirty seconds to one minute)

● Lie on your front, with your arms bent and the palms of your hands resting on the floor close to your body at shoulder level. Your forehead should be touching the floor.

● Push your legs slightly back, raising your feet on your toes, and bring your forehead slightly forward to stretch your spinal column. (1)

● Push your chin along the floor and slowly bend your head backwards.

Cobra pose (1)

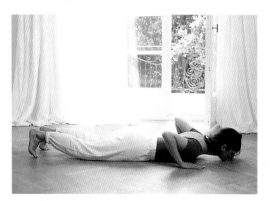

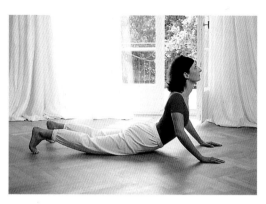

● Lift your head and upper body, pressing your hands to the floor. Your navel should still be touching the floor (2).

● Stay in this position for a few seconds: you will feel an intense stretching sensation in your chest and back. Breathe slowly and evenly.

● Let your upper body slide slowly downwards, touch the floor with your chin then move your head so that your forehead touches the floor.

● Relax comfortably for a few breaths then repeat the exercise.

Cobra pose (2)

Spinal twist
(about one minute)

● Sit upright on the floor with your legs outstretched in front of you. Bend your right knee, placing the foot flat on the floor. Bring your knee close to your upper body, keeping your left leg straight.

● Place your right hand behind you for support, then curl your left arm around the outside of your right knee and grasp the knee with your hand (1).

● The pose has an even more intense effect if you place your right foot on the far side of your left leg. (2).

Spinal twist (1)

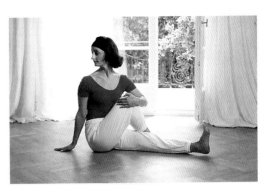

Spinal twist (2)

● Staying in this pose, breathe in, lift your thorax and stretch your spinal column upwards.

● As you breathe out, turn your body and head to the right, moving from the base of the spine.

● Breathe calmly and evenly. Remain sitting in this position for a few moments before slowly straightening up.

● Repeat the spinal twist on the other side.

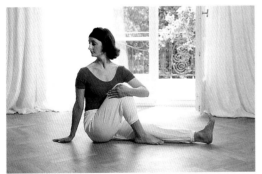

Corpse Pose
(one to two minutes)

● Lie down flat so that your whole back is touching the floor.
● Stretch your legs, with your feet relaxed and pointing outwards (see photograph below).
● Relax your head, neck, shoulders and hips. Rest your arms loosely by your sides, with the palms of your hands upwards.
● Close your eyes and breathe gently and evenly.

Corpse pose

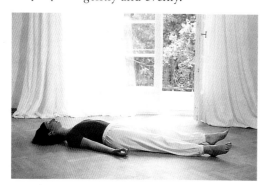

Breathing exercises
(Pranayama)

Ayurveda attaches great importance to breathing, which has a profound but subtle effect on our well-being. For this reason, breathing exercises are among the basic methods of balancing the doshas.

To achieve a correct rhythm of breathing, Ayurveda teaches you to breathe alternately through each nostril. The two most important effects of this and of rhythmic, regular breathing are:

● Firstly, a calming influence on the nervous system – after breathing exercises you will feel noticeably more relaxed.
● Secondly, the Pranayama breathing technique reconciles the opposite sides of our nature. According to ancient Indian belief, the right respiratory channel, in other words the right nostril, is connected to our active rational side. The left respiratory channel, or left nostril, is a link with our passive emotional side. The two qualities are the opposite poles of our existence. Through alternate nostril breathing we can bring the two sides into harmony, so that neither one is noticeably weaker than the other.

Harmonizing the two sides of our nature

Breathing exercises

For five minutes every morning and evening, practise breathing in the following way. To make sure your breathing is regular, it may help to count as you do the exercise: breathe in, out and rest to a slow count of 5.

● Sit upright but comfortably on a chair, or cross-legged on the floor. Make sure your chest and abdomen are not constricted by tight clothing.
● Close your eyes and inhale then exhale deeply a few times. Focus all your concentration on your breathing.
● Place your right thumb against your right nostril, pressing lightly to close the airway (1).
● Breathe out slowly through your open left nostril, then rest for a moment. After a few seconds your body will demand that you breathe in.
● Breathe in through your left nostril, then pinch it closed with the middle and fourth fingers of your right hand. At the same time, release your right nostril and let the air you are holding escape. (2). Breathe out slowly through the right nostril. Then hold your breath for a moment.

Breathe in a relaxed way

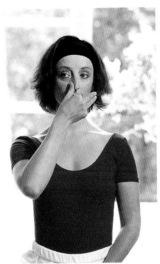

Breathing exercise (1) – hand position

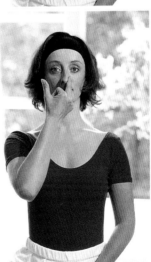

Breathing exercise (2) – hand position

- Breathe in through your right nostril, then press it closed again with your thumb.
- Breathe out through the left nostril.
- Repeat the breathing sequence, alternating between the left and right nostrils.
To finish the exercise, inhale through your left nostril, then remove your finger so that both airways are clear and breathe out through both nostrils.
- Sit quietly for a minute or two, breathing regularly with your eyes closed, to allow the exercise to take effect.

Important

Avoid any kind of tension as you breathe – it should all happen easily and without strain.

If you start to feel dizzy, rest for a moment, open your eyes and breathe normally. As soon as you feel comfortable again, continue with the exercise.

Try not to control your breathing, do not hold your breath or count the number of breaths. Carry out the exercise in as natural and relaxed a way as possible.

Meditation to cleanse and calm the spirit

One of the most important Ayurvedic methods of permanently stabilizing the doshas is meditation. In the same way that Panchakarma purifies the body, the spirit must also be cleansed.

Practitioners of Ayurveda believe that waste products and impurities produced by the body also have their mental and emotional counterparts. Greed, envy, jealousy, compulsive behaviour and constant self-doubt are a few examples of the negative emotions that often trouble us. If these emotions or attitudes are not resolved or overcome, they build up inside us and have the same effect as chemical stress hormones. Such negative mental or emotional patterns are known as *emotional ama*.

Meditation is one of the most constructive ways of ridding the spirit of ama and deeply relaxing the body. The spirit provides the starting point from which to harmonize the doshas.

It has been known for thousands of years that meditation can have a remarkably positive impact on

Meditation for deep relaxation

a person. This has now been proven by scientific research. There is evidence that regular meditation has a positive influence on physical bodily processes such as the heart, circulatory and respiratory functions, which in turn reduces the risk of disease.

Likewise, there is evidence that meditation has a beneficial effect on the emotions. Improved spiritual well-being helps to conquer negative reactions and transform them into positive personality traits, feelings of self-worth, and a tolerant attitude.

A simple meditation exercise

Ideally, you should meditate immediately after completing the Pranayama breathing exercise, since rhythmic breathing is an important precondition for meditation. Meditate for 10 to 15 minutes.

- Sit on a chair or cross-legged on the floor. The lotus position – if you can manage it – is perfect for meditation.

Emotional well-being through meditation

- It is important that you sit comfortably, with your back straight.

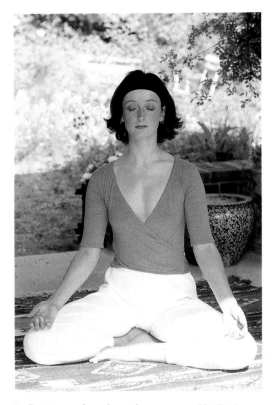

- Rest your hands, palms upwards, on your thighs. Your hands should be cupped, but relaxed (see photograph above). Lay a small cushion on your lap, if this is more comfortable for your hands.

Meditation exercise

- Close your eyes and breathe in and out five times. Aim to reach a state of inner calm.

- Continue to breathe evenly while you focus your mind on the words: "let go". If other thoughts enter your mind, just let them drift.

Let your mind wander

● Do not try to hold on to any particular thought and avoid any attempt to evaluate what is going on inside you. Just let your mind wander.

● Breathe slowly and calmly. With each breath think: "let go". Allow your mind and body to relax completely. Focus your attention inwards.

● Do not attempt to direct or control your thoughts – just continue to think of the words "let go". After a while, consciously breathe more deeply.

● Open your eyes and take a little time to rest and work through your feelings.

Important

If you want a thorough grounding in meditation techniques, you will need practical help and advice from an experienced meditation teacher. The exercise described is not intended as an introduction to the practice of meditation. It is designed to give you a first impression, as well as the chance to try out the method at home in your own time.

Training the senses

Our five senses enable us to find our way through the world. On the obvious level, our senses allow us to perceive external objects through sight, hearing, touch, taste and smell. In a less obvious way, our senses help us to organize our thoughts and feelings.

In Ayurveda, full use of the senses is considered an important prerequisite of good health, since our sensory impressions can influence the workings of our mind and emotions. Smells, colours, sounds, the objects we touch and the food we taste all influence balance, and can stabilize the equilibrium of the doshas or restore harmony when they are disturbed. Educating the senses, therefore, is effectively another form of healing.

According to Ayurvedic theory, different senses are developed to different levels in each constitutional type. Vata types are characterized by clear senses of hearing and taste. Pitta types have strong visual perception. Kapha types take special delight in smells and tastes.

Strong sensory perception

Aromatherapy

In Ayurvedic sensory training, aromatherapy using plant fragrances is one of the main methods of influencing our physical, mental and emotional processes.

In aromatherapy, smells penetrate the area of the brain responsible for the emotions and important physical functions via special cells. Ayurveda uses this healing power in various ways.

Since our senses of smell and taste are closely related, Ayurveda recommends that we season food with specific herbs and spices (see pages 85, 87 and 89). This enables their distinctive aromas to develop within the body.

Herbs and spices

As well as herbs and spices, essential oils are used as natural remedies in Ayurvedic aromatherapy. Their fragrant message can be transmitted to the internal organs, either through the skin – by massage, for example – or through inhalation.

Healing with essential oils

Which aromas are right for you?

A selection of herbs and spices to benefit different constitutional types can be found in the chapter on diet (see page 71).

The table below suggests oils which are suitable for balancing the three doshas. When choosing an oil for yourself:

Oils to balance the doshas

● Be guided by your main dosha and by the way you feel at the time: use the oil that will balance your endangered or disturbed dosha.

● Trust your own sense of smell. Test the oils before buying, since the oil to which you are spontaneously attracted will be exactly right for your purpose.

Vata can be harmonized with a blend of sweet and acidic aromas, such as basil, orange, geranium and cloves.

Pitta balance is improved by a mixture of fresh, sweet perfumes, like sandalwood, rose, mint, cinnamon or jasmine.

Kapha equilibrium is promoted by spicy, earthy fragrances, including juniper, eucalyptus, camphor, cloves or marjoram.

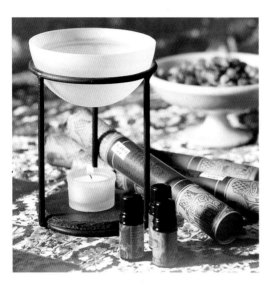

may be different from a mixture intended for massage: be sure to get the appropriate preparation for your needs.

Colour therapy

We cannot live without light and colour. Colour delights the eye and senses and can help create whatever atmosphere you desire. The colours of your home, your clothes, and even the food you eat, have a subtle influence on your quality of life and your prevailing mood.

Colours influence your quality of life

For this reason, colour therapy has a major role in the Ayurvedic sensory education programme. Each colour produces different vibrations in the body, which in turn restore or stabilize the balance between vata, pitta and kapha.

The therapy is based on the seven colours of the rainbow (see illustration on page 62), which are correlated with the five elements and the three doshas.

Inhalation

Take care when choosing oil for a burner

To inhale a blend of fragrances, you will need an oil burner, or simply a little bowl that you can stand over a flame. Depending on the size of the room, sprinkle between 10 and 15 drops of aromatic oil into the bowl, and top up with warm water. You can inhale an aroma for half an hour or longer each day, according to your needs.

Essential oils are available from pharmacies and health food shops. You can also obtain oil mixtures suited to your constitutional type from Ayurvedic practitioners. An oil mixture suitable for inhalation

Everyday colour therapy

As with essential oils, you can choose colours that are suited to your main dosha and to how you are feeling at any particular

The influence of colours

Red is associated with blood. It gives it its colour and promotes the formation of red corpuscles. Red also produces heat, stimulates circulation, determines skin colour and supplies energy to the nerves and bone marrow. It facilitates blood flow, dilating and unblocking the blood vessels. Disturbances of the vata or kapha doshas are pacified by red, but pitta types should avoid this colour, or use it with caution.

Colours produce vibrations

Orange, like red and yellow, is a warm colour, bolstering sexual energy and stimulating kidney function. The effects of orange are constructive, fortifying, positive and healthy. Psychologically, it is antidepressant and uplifting. Orange has a beneficial influence on vata and kapha imbalances.

Yellow represents repose and instils feelings of weightlessness and serenity. This colour has a stabilizing effect at the deepest level. It influences glandular function, activating the mucous membranes and promoting secretion. In cases of stomach and liver complaints, yellow stimulates elimination. Nevertheless, incorrect use can lead to pitta disturbance in the small intestine. Without a thorough diagnosis, pitta types should avoid the warm colours – red, orange and yellow – or use them with discretion. However, yellow is an excellent means of stabilizing excess vata and kapha.

Green represents regeneration, equilibrium and harmony, and has a calming influence on the mind and spirit. At the same time, green promotes our powers of concentration. Used excessively, green can lead to pitta disturbance in the production and flow of bile.

Pale green combines the qualities and effects of its component colours: yellow and green.

Blue represents tranquillity, space and coolness. Its effects are to reduce, corrode, inhibit and contract. Blue relieves disturbances in skin pigmentation and has a positive effect on pitta imbalances. Vata and kapha types, however, should use blue with caution.

Colours influence moods

Purple, like blue, is a cold colour. It has a balancing effect, as it diminishes coldness but restricts heat. Purple affects the central nervous system and promotes sleep. It has a pacifying, relaxing and even slightly hypnotic influence. Purple is extremely useful in treating pitta and kapha imbalances, but it can be harmful to vata if incorrectly used.

The Ayurvedic approach to health and healing

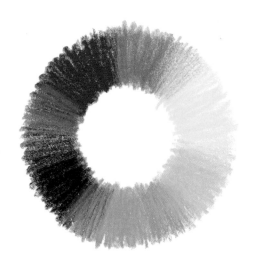

Colours of the spectrum

• You can choose food according to colour. Select fruit and vegetables to match the colours that meet your needs.

Music therapy

Ayurvedic sensory training is based on listening to certain melodies taken from the *Gandharva Veda*, which forms part of ancient vedic literature. The name Gandharva Veda, means "the knowledge of sounds".

According to ancient vedic tradition, hearing particular sounds influences body, mind and spirit. In the same way that the doshas respond to tastes, colours and smells, specific melodies, pieces of music, sounds and tone colours can stabilize or disturb vata, pitta and kapha.

The stabilizing effect of music

time. You can carry out your own colour therapy programme in various ways:

• Spend some time looking at colourful pictures and flowers, or wear brightly coloured clothes.

• Another possibility is to relax in a "coloured bath". Choose bath salts or bubble bath according to their colour and perfume. You might, for example, enjoy the bluish purple colour of a lavender-scented bath, or orange bath water with the fragrance of orange blossom, or yellow water perfumed with lemon.

Time and season: living in tune with nature

The human being is a microcosm arranged exactly like the universe, the macrocosm. This assumption is at the intellectual root of the Ayurvedic philosophy of life. Accordingly, the tridoshas influence not only our organs and spiritual well-being, but are also bound up with the recurring, natural rhythms of the day, the year and the human life-span.

This theory, which Indian sages skilled in the art of healing believed thousands of years ago, is now an aspect of *chronobiology*, a specialized branch of biology which researches the relationship between life events and the natural laws of chronology.

One of the most important results of chronobiological research has been the discovery of the connection between the natural rhythm of the cosmos and human biorhythms:

Cosmic rhythm = biorhythm

● Degrees of light and darkness, heat and cold, dryness and wetness differ according to the time of day

and the season of the year. All biological systems – humans, animals, plants – are subject to these changes. Consequently, we and all living things around us are constantly adapting to varying conditions.

Changing patterns of life

● You may find that you can work with the greatest concentration at a particular time of day; you may feel slightly depressed in winter; or you may have to fight off feelings of tiredness in spring. All these are examples of how daily and annual rhythms influence our lives.

■ Ayurveda recognizes the influence that the rhythms of nature have on all forms of life. Central to Ayurvedic belief is the theory that, if we allow ourselves to be guided by the natural conditions around us, we can regulate the balance of our inner energies in a natural way. The doshas gradually adapt to the rhythms they are most closely related to, and so achieve their counterpart, or "likeness", in nature.

Harmonizing with the rhythm of time

A healthy, natural life is one that is attuned to biological rhythms.

If you make the necessary adjustments to enable you to live in harmony with the rhythms of the day, the year and the stage you have reached in your own life cycle, you will increase your ability to function efficiently, and improve your general well-being.

The rhythm of the day

Two cycles

Ayurveda divides the 24 hours of the day and night into two principal cycles. These, in turn, are composed of three phases, and each phase is governed by one dosha:

First cycle	Dosha
06.00 to 10.00 hours	Kapha
10.00 to 14.00 hours	Pitta
14.00 to 18.00 hours	Vata

Second cycle	Dosha
18.00 to 22.00 hours	Kapha
22.00 to 02.00 hours	Pitta
02.00 to 06.00 hours	Vata

Kapha phase

● Kapha energy is at its height from the first light of dawn. The morning hours between 6.00 and 10 .00 are, in Ayurvedic terms, the period in which the body summons up the energy to tackle the events of the day. We are advised to use this time of day for purification rituals and generally to attend to our needs.

Pitta phase

● The pitta phase is the time around midday, when we are most active and have the strongest appetite. Pitta is responsible for the fire within the body and for converting food into energy (see page 18). For this reason it is vital to eat the main meal of the day at this time, when we are best able to digest efficiently.

Vata phase

● The pitta phase now gives way to the vata phase. We are at our most creative and communicative between 14.00 and 18.00 in the afternoon. Our motor skills are also enhanced during the vata phase. Nevertheless, this is a good time to take a regular, relaxing break, to avoid increased activity turning into negative stress.

Second cycle

The second daily cycle repeats the kapha, pitta, vata sequence, but the regulatory mechanisms of the doshas have different objectives.

● Kapha makes us feel lethargic and tired in the evening. Pitta now uses its internal fire not only to digest food, but also to keep the body warm during sleep. And instead of speeding up our thought processes, in the early hours of the morning vata gives us vivid dreams.

The second cycle brings the day to an end, completing the 24-hour sequence.

Morning routine: between 6.00 and 8.00 hours
● Let your "internal clock" awaken you naturally, without an alarm.
● Drink a glass or a few sips of warm water to encourage morning bowel movement (page 35).
● Allow plenty of time to empty your bladder and bowels.
● Clean your teeth thoroughly.
● Oil and massage your body with sesame oil (page 37).
● Take a warm bath or shower.
● Perform the Salute to the Sun (page 44) and/or the yoga exercise sequence (page 50), and the breathing exercises (page 54).
● Meditation (page 56).
● Eat a light, unhurried breakfast.
● If time allows, take a 15 to 30 minute walk.

Lunch: between 12.00 and 13.00 hours
● Eat an early lunch, as your main meal of the day.
● After eating, sit quietly for 5 minutes.
● Take a 5 to 10-minute walk to help your digestion.
● Meditate in the late afternoon.

Living in tune with nature

Evening meal: between 18.00 and 19.00
● Eat a light dinner.
● After eating, sit quietly for 5 minutes.
● Take a 15-minute walk to help your digestion.

Bedtime: between 21.30 and 22.30
● Avoid strenuous activity in the evening
● Try to go to bed between the recommended times (at least three hours after dinner)
● Do not read or watch television in bed

The daily routine

Observing the Ayurvedic rhythms of the day is an important step towards bringing health and harmony into our daily lives.

In Ayurvedic practice, certain routine tasks are carried out at particular times of day. The box on page 65 outlines an Ayurvedic routine for a range of daily activities. If you regularly follow this routine, you will find after a time that you are able to make the most of your energy potential: you will be living and working according to, rather than against, your nature.

Live according to your nature

The rhythm of the year

According to Ayurvedic belief, we are influenced not only by the rhythm of the day, but also by the changing seasons. In the same way that the doshas correspond to times of the day, they also have their special times of year:

● The kapha season extends from mid-March until mid-June, more or less parallel to what we call spring.

● The pitta season runs from the middle of June until mid-October, corresponding to summer and early autumn.

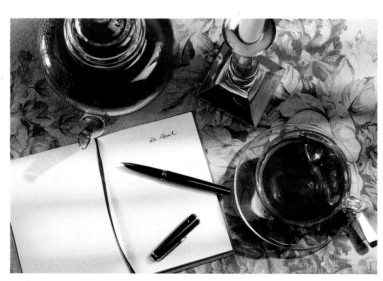

Make time to keep a diary – one of the best ways to combat stress

The influence of the changing seasons

● The vata season begins in mid-October and continues until mid-March, equivalent to late autumn and winter.

These three Ayurvedic seasons must always take account of local conditions. For example, in India, where the climate is different to that of western Europe, there are six seasons in all. Ultimately, this means that it is not the calendar but the actual weather conditions that decide which dosha applies.

Sensitivity to the weather

What we understand by the expression "sensitive to the weather" – a discernible personal reaction to particular climatic conditions – is a concept that has been recognized in Ayurveda for thousands of years. The characteristics of vata, pitta and kapha are matched by different weather characteristics and the three doshas are extremely sensitive to sudden changes in weather conditions – irrespective of the time of year at which they occur, since the prevailing weather triggers specific doshic responses.

When we experience a particular kind of weather

which shares the same characteristics as a particular dosha, the effect can often be felt very clearly.

Vata is closely related to such conditions as cold, dryness, lightness and mobility. Vata accumulates during cold, windy weather. When a vata person is exposed for too long to these conditions, the result may be agitation and general malaise. Pitta increases on hot, humid summer days, while kapha is intensified by cold and damp, or snow.

Keeping an eye on the weather

The yearly routine

As well as observing a daily routine, Ayurveda also recommends a seasonal programme. The guiding principle is:

▶ Be particularly on your guard during the season corresponding to your constitutional type – kapha types in spring, pitta types in summer, and vata types in winter. Your doshas can all too easily become unbalanced during these periods of the year. To ensure that they do not suffer imbalance, observe the following rules:

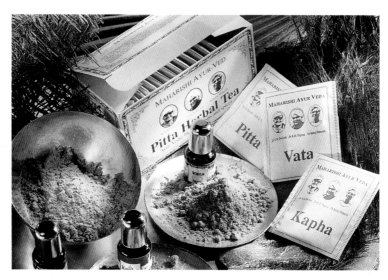

Teas, spices and oils for each dosha type

Balancing the doshas

● Only expose yourself in "small doses" to the kind of weather corresponding to your main dosha.

● Follow a diet suited to your constitution (see the following chapter).

● Add suitable spices to your meals, and regularly drink tea blends appropriate to your type.

● Follow the daily routine set out on page 65.

● In spring – the Kapha season – undertake a Panchakarma, a purification cure, to eliminate waste products and toxins.

● Respect your constitution and your personal needs if you choose a holiday destination with extreme climatic conditions.

The rhythm of life

Ayurveda recognises a third important cycle relating to the three doshas. Like the day and the year, our entire life span is divided into three stages, whose characteristics correspond to those of vata, pitta and kapha.

The three stages of life

● The first stage of life is one of growth and development both physically and intellectually. Accordingly, the period from birth to the age of years about 30 is known as the kapha phase.

● The pitta phase occurs between the ages of 30 and 60. This is the period in which we apply our acquired skills and knowledge, and so is the most productive stage of our lives.

● From the age of about 60, a process of physical decline and transformation begins. As we pass from our active, productive phase into one in which we become physically more passive, more activity starts to take place on the intellectual level. This is the vata period.

Staying youthful in old age

Listening to our bodies

Whichever stage of our lives we are at, we have to learn to listen to the voices of our bodies in order to maintain health and harmony.

The science of long, healthy life teaches us how to get in touch with the inner wisdom of the body. It also shows how the completely natural process of ageing can be delayed. In Ayurvedic theory, the notion of ageing is an "intellectual error", since it only thinks of people in terms of their physical condition.

Ageing: an "intellectual error"

To prolong life, we must first of all correct this false assumption. If we let ourselves be guided not by our biological clock but by the freshness and capability of our minds, we become in a sense ageless. The physical result of this mental attitude is actually to slow down the body's ageing process. Ayurveda regards a hundred years as the normal human life expectancy.

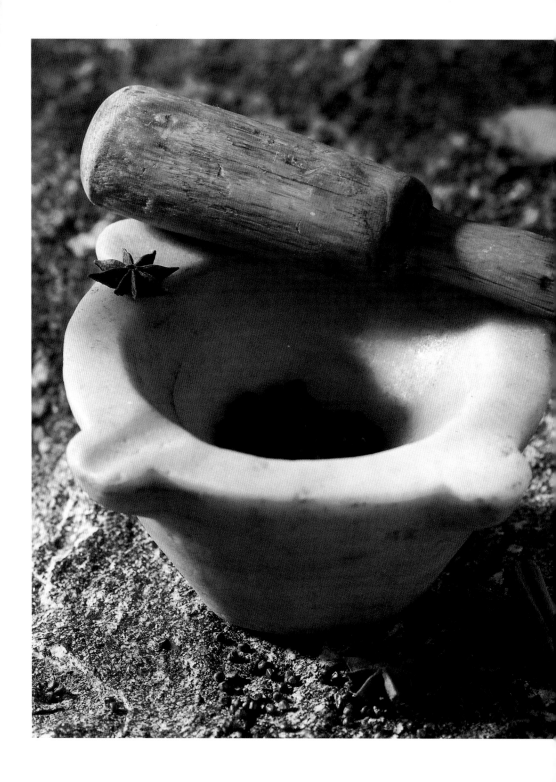

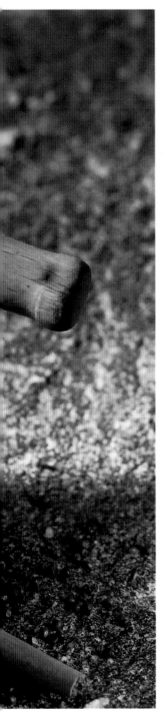

Eating what the body needs

"Food provides the living being with the strength to live."
Charaka Samhita (6. Jh. v. Chr.)

Ayurveda attaches great importance to a healthy, balanced diet, for good food, eaten in tranquillity at the right time of day, is a medicine in itself. Food balances the doshas, increasing resistance to illness and maintaining well-being.

However, the Ayurvedic concept of nutrition in no way prescribes a strict diet. You simply pay attention to your body's needs. All those things you enjoy eating are also exactly what you need to retain the balance of body, mind and emotions. Find out what Ayurveda means by the "right" diet in the following chapter.

The right diet is the best medicine

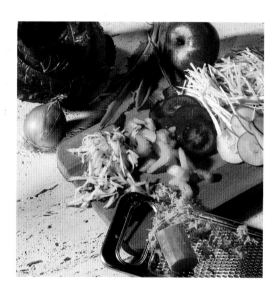

What we eat and how much, how we prepare food, how much time we spend eating, and our emotional state while we are eating – all these are factors that determine whether we are eating correctly or incorrectly, healthily or unhealthily. Ayurveda looks on food as a natural medicine: a trained practitioner will only prescribe drugs or medicinal herbs when diet alone fails to promote healing.

Efficient digestion is just as important as the type and quality of food. Even healthy, nourishing food can damage our health if not properly digested. It results in a build-up of ama – waste products, toxins and undigested food.

Ayurvedic dietary recommendations take account of your personality, your natural constitution, current state of health and physical, mental and emotional needs.

Dietary recommen-dations

Eating with all the senses

Many ailments of the modern world are directly or indirectly linked to poor nutrition. Obesity, digestive problems and deficiency symptoms are just some of the manifestations of incorrect eating habits. And although western dieticians are constantly giving advice about what we should or should not eat, it appears that this knowledge has not so far helped a great deal: the number of diet-related illnesses seems to be ever-increasing.

Sensory perception of food

Western diets have us counting calories and carbohydrates, measuring fats and proteins, and analysing our vitamin and mineral intake. Ayurveda is less concerned with such things. Although Ayurveda does recommend food combining, the focal point of the Ayurvedic concept of nutrition is each person's own sensory perception.

Our senses are unable to detect all the properties of food. We know very well that an orange contains a lot of vitamin C, but we can neither taste, smell nor see it – to us it is an abstract idea. In Ayurvedic practice our *subjective* response to eating a particular food is considered to be much more important than the objective contents of the item. When you eat an orange you taste its characteristic flavour, which is something you can both perceive and enjoy.

Throughout your life, you will probably have developed preferences for certain foods and aversions to others. It is this, no doubt, that dictates your choice of food, rather than what nutritionists tell you about them. This is entirely in accord with Ayurvedic theory, which holds that eating is first and foremost a sensory experience, dictated neither by intellect nor by dietary charts.

Eating – an experience for the senses

■ The value of any food depends on the individual's tolerance, current needs, and personal likes and dislikes. The foods you enjoy, the ones you find particularly tasty and those that make you feel good after eating them, these are the best foods – and therefore medicine – for your body.

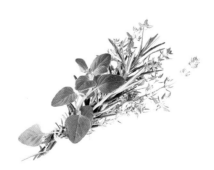

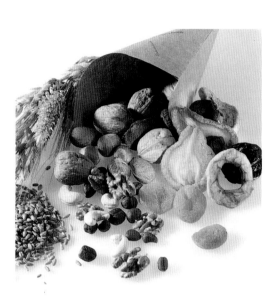

Wholesome
food can
heal

The six tastes

When we eat, a great deal of our response depends on taste. If you like the flavour of a food you will eat it with relish. The reaction of your taste buds is purely subjective. Some people, for example, love hot and spicy food, while others simply cannot stand to eat highly seasoned dishes. It leaves them with a numbed mouth and an upset stomach.

The physical characteristics of the food that we eat – whether it lies heavily on the stomach, whether it is fatty, oily, or dry, whether it warms or cools the body – are also decisive factors. These different characteristics, known as *gunas*, work in distinctive ways on the doshas and are in large part responsible for how we react to different foods.

However, the three vital energies receive their most crucial messages from the *rasas*, or kinds of taste. As well as the five types of taste that we in the West recognize – sweet, sour, salty, pungent and bitter – Ayurveda includes a sixth taste: astringent.

Ideally, every meal should include all six rasas, as this will ensure a genuinely balancing effect on the three vital energies of vata, pitta and kapha.

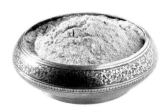

Rock salt

The six tastes

The following examples show how the six tastes apply in specific foods:

Sweet
(Madhur)

Grains such as wheat, barley, rye and oats; fruits such as oranges, bananas, pears, grapes and figs; vegetables such as cucumber, onions, cabbage, lentils and peas; nuts such as walnuts, peanuts and coconut; oils such as sesame, castor, sunflower and olive oil; sweet dairy products; butter, ghee and honey; meat; rice; potatoes; sugar.

Sour
(Amla)

Dairy products such as yoghurt, cheese and products fermented with lactic acid; fruits such as rosehips, pomegranate, morello cherries, lemon; vinegar.

Salty
(Lavan)

All types of salt, including sea and rock salt (Ayurveda recommends rock salt for seasoning).

Pungent
(Katu)

Spices and herbs such as pepper, chilli, basil, oregano, marjoram, rosemary, thyme, nutmeg and caraway; radish, sweet peppers, ginger, parsley, dill and camomile; essential oils.

Bitter
(Tikta)

Salad leaves such as radicchio, dandelion, rocket, green lettuce; green leaf vegetables such as spinach, Brussels sprouts and Swiss chard; bitter herbs and spices such as sorrel, fenugreek, yellow gentian, centaury, nettles, tobacco and horse chestnut; rhubarb.

Astringent
(Kasay)

Pulses such as beans, mung beans, green peas, chick peas, lentils; vegetables such as cauliflower, broccoli, chicory, fennel, asparagus, aubergines, savoy cabbage, celery; fruits such as apples and pears.

Characteristics of staple foods

As well as the six tastes, Ayurveda also distinguishes between six characteristics, arranged in contrasting pairs:

Heavy or light:

Wheat is heavy, barley is light; beef is heavy, chicken or turkey is light; cheese is heavy, skimmed milk is light.

Oily or dry:

Milk is oily, honey is dry; soy beans are oily, lentils are dry; coconut is oily, cabbage is dry.

Hot or cold:

Pepper is hot, mint is cold; honey is hot, sugar is cold; eggs are hot, milk is cold.

The right diet is the best medicine

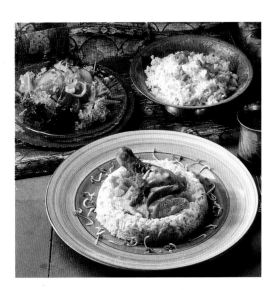

A balanced meal: roasted chicken with rice and salad

Which diet is best for you?

Your choice of food should be guided by the following basic principle:

▶ Eat food that reduces the energy of your predominant dosha and fortifies your secondary or subsidiary doshas.

For example: If you are a kapha type, your menu should include mainly foods which pacify your kapha, your main dosha, and which strengthen vata and pitta, your secondary for subsidiary doshas.

This way of eating might sound complicated at first, until you realise that the knowledge of which foods are needed to balance your doshas is already stored away in your body.

As soon as you learn to pay greater attention to your body's needs you will, for example, insist on warm, comforting food when you feel cold. If you are a vata type you might add more salt to your meals, since people of this type need not fear health problems if they sometimes take a little too much salt.

At the same time, always bear in mind that your meals should, as far as possible, include all six tastes. Roast chicken with rice and salad is a good example of a balanced midday meal. It contains all six tastes as follows: bitter and astringent (salad); sour (salad dressing with vinegar or lemon juice); salty and pungent (chicken seasoned with salt, pepper and curry powder); and sweet (rice).

■ In Ayurvedic terms, a "balanced" daily diet is one containing all six rasas or tastes. However, you should also take account of the characteristics or gunas of your chosen foods, because the doshas react to the properties of both rasas and gunas.

A balanced diet

Doshas	Tastes (Rasas)	Characteristics (Gunas)	
Vata-pacifying	sweet, sour, salty	heavy, oily, hot	Choose
Vata-strengthening	pungent, bitter, astringent	light, dry, cold	according to
			your type
Pitta-pacifying	sweet, bitter, astringent	cold, heavy, dry	
Pitta-strengthening	pungent, sour, salty	hot, light, oily	
Kapha-pacifying	pungent, bitter, astringent	light, dry, hot	
Kapha-strengthening	sweet, sour, salty	heavy, oily, cold	

Food as natural therapy

A healthy diet balances vata, pitta and kapha, and keeps them permanently in equilibrium. In this way, our daily food intake provides a highly effective form of therapy. The right food will pacify doshic excess and eliminate any insufficiency.

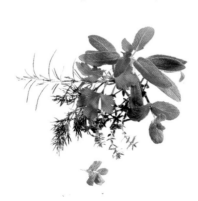

Dietary supplements

As an extension of the Ayurvedic principle of nutritional balance, there are also a number of supplements which can enable us to derive even greater benefit from the food we eat. Known as *rasayanas*, which translates as "putting in the essence of life", they include specific medicinal herbs and minerals which singly or in combination help to maximise health and prolong life.

Only a few of the innumerable rasayanas known in India are commonly available in the West. Those that are include gotu kola and ginseng recommended for vata types; aloe vera, comfrey and saffron for pitta types; and elecampane and honey for kapha types. (Although honey is not a medicinal herb it is

The right diet is the best medicine

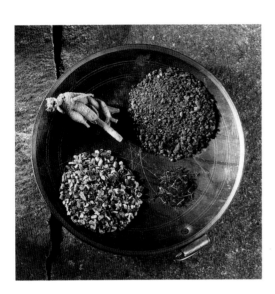

Ayurvedic medicinal herbs

Vegetarian or not?

In essence, Ayurveda advocates being vegetarian because a meatless diet is regarded as the healthiest. Nevertheless, Ayurveda does offer advice for meat-eaters on which meat is best suited to the different constitutional types.

A vegetarian regime, or one in which meat is reduced, plays a vital role in the treatment of some ailments. Ayurveda would recommend:

regarded as the purest product of the plant world.)

A special rasayana recommended by Ayurvedic practitioners is chyavan prash, which is sometimes seen as amrit kalash. This preparation of herbs and fruit is blended according to a recipe thousands of years old, and can be obtained in the West in paste or tablet form. It is sometimes recommended that people taking a panchakarma purification cure should take this rasayana twice daily. Regular use is said to have an intense strengthening and harmonizing effect, building up resistance to disease and slowing the process of ageing.

● If you regularly eat meat, start taking smaller portions. As often as possible, replace red meat (beef, pork, veal) with poultry or fish.

After a while, you will find it becomes easier and easier to eat less or even no meat.

Gradually cut down on meat

The importance of good digestion

Nearly all of us suffer from digestive problems: flatulence, bloating, constipation, heartburn or belching are a few the common indications that all is not entirely well with the digestive tract. Unfortunately, we usually pay little attention to these everyday disorders. They either cure themselves or many people reach for pills to combat the irritation.

Foundation of good health

From the Ayurvedic point of view, however, even trivial digestive problems are the forerunners of a variety of ailments. A good digestion is the foundation of a long and healthy life and for this reason, whatever your constitutional type, you should pay attention to your digestion. Different types are prone to different digestive problems:

How each type digests

● Vata types are prone to irregular digestion. Pitta types sometimes digest too quickly. Kapha types often suffer from slow and difficult digestion.

Agni – the fire of digestion

Agni is the Ayurvedic term applied to our power of digestion. The word means "fire", or in a biological sense, digestive energy. A second meaning is the "flame of life", which burns brightly when we are in good health and is extinguished when we die. *Agni* relates to our entire way of life, in which diet is the most important factor.

Lifestyle governs *agni*

Different demands are made on the digestive fire according to the type, quality and quantity of our food. Eating too much or too often, heavy meals, unhealthy food or too much protein taken in the evening can all diminish the fire so the "flame of life" loses its intensity. Moreover, eating the main meal in the evening weakens the fire, as does reading, watching television or quarrelling while eating.

■ *Agni*, the "fire of digestion", is one of the body's most important functions. It ensures that we digest our food efficiently, that each body cell absorbs the nourishment necessary to life, and that all waste products are burnt off, leaving no harmful residues. Incorrect diet and unhealthy eating behaviour are two **Disruptive factors** disruptive factors that can diminish *agni*, which in turn may lead to serious stomach and intestinal complaints.

Improving your digestion

Ayurveda recommends particular foods, spices and herbs to improve the quality of the *agni* in the different constitutional types. The following substances are a completely natural way of stimulating the appetite, promoting healthy digestion and eliminating *ama*, the body's waste products.

Stimulating your agni ● Ginger helps stabilize *agni* in every constitutional type. Fresh ginger is best, but the ground variety is also good. It can serve as a seasoning, or be made into tea. A cup of ginger tea before meals increases

appetite, while sipping the tea during or after the meal aids digestion.

● Ghee, or clarified butter, is one of the mainstays of the Ayurvedic diet (see page 83). It strengthens *agni*, without inflaming pitta – the fiery element. Ghee is very useful in balancing pitta, and also helpful in reducing excess kapha. Ayurveda recommends

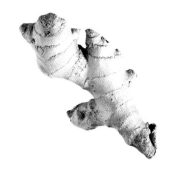

Ginger root

the use of ghee as a tasty alternative to normal butter. To improve digestion, sprinkle a teaspoonful of ghee over your food. You can buy ghee in health food shops, or specialist Indian stores, or you can make your own. Ghee will keep for several months if stored in a cool dry place, so you can make it in quite a large quantity. To make ghee, put 1 kg of unsalted butter in a large heavy pan and heat slowly, stirring all the time, until it is melted. Turn up the heat until the butter froths, then turn the heat down as low as possible and leave to simmer gently, uncovered, for about half and hour. When the butter is clear enough for you to see the bottom of the pan, strain it through a fine sieve or cloth into a clean jar or other container then leave to cool.

● Other spices that will generally improve *agni* include black pepper, cloves, cardamom, horseradish, cayenne pepper, mustard and cinnamon. Pitta types should only use these spices sparingly, as they slightly increase pitta.

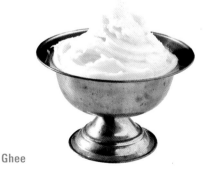

Ghee

Ayurveda's 10 golden rules for a healthy diet

Here are some general guidelines to help you plan your daily diet. They apply to all constitutional types.

1 Eat in a calm, pleasant atmosphere and think about what you are eating. Do not work, read or watch television while you eat, and always sit down to meals.

Eat in a calm atmosphere

2 Always choose wholesome foods that both taste and look good.

3 Try to eat at the same time each day. Do not bolt your food, but chew it thoroughly. Eat to only three-quarters of your capacity: stop when you are full, but not over-full.

4 Allow three to six hours between meals to give yourself time to digest the previous meal properly. If you are very hungry (as opposed to merely fancying a snack), this is a sure sign that your body needs more food. Nevertheless, do not eat if you are not hungry.

Leave intervals between meals

5 Sip water or juice with your meals. Drinks should not be ice-cold as this inhibits digestion. Ideally, drink hot water, perhaps with a little ginger added.

6 Choose fresh foods, which are preferably produced locally. Three-quarters of your menu should consist of warm, freshly-prepared food, and the remaining quarter of salad and other cold ingredients. This is because warm, cooked dishes are easier to digest than cold, uncooked food. A warm, suitably seasoned meal containing a little fat is the best choice. If possible, avoid reheated food.

Eat easily digestible foods in the evening

7 At the evening meal, avoid sour dairy products, animal protein and raw ingredients. All of these are hard to digest and at this time of day your digestive "fire" burns dimly.

8 If possible, always eat your main meal at midday, since your digestion functions most efficiently between 12.00 and 13.00 hours. Take only a light meal in the evening.

9 Always take time to relax for a few minutes after eating and before you resume work or study.

Relax after eating

10 The surest way to eat well is to trust your own body, which will demand what it needs. Poor or incorrect eating habits, or an existing doshic imbalance, can, of course, lead to unhealthy cravings. Check your own diet and try to integrate the Ayurvedic guidelines for eating into your daily life.

Trust your own body

A diet for your constitutional type

Perhaps you have already wondered why you are not keen on certain vegetables or salads, but can eat vast quantities of fruit, or prefer why you prefer cooked meals, while cold or raw foods have little appeal. You may also have noticed that you have a preference for certain foods in summer, but enjoy different foods in the cold winter months.

Ayurveda can easily explain all of this. Each of us intuitively eats according to our constitutional type and the time of year. As pointed out on page 74, certain tastes and characteristics of food can either pacify or strengthen the doshas.

Balancing the doshas

▶ Pay heed to the signals your body gives you, since it will crave a particular taste or characteristic to keep its doshas in equilibrium.

To ensure that your diet is in harmony with your inner nature, you must first and foremost observe these two basic dietary guideliness:

Dietary guidelines

● Choose foods that balance or pacify your predominant dosha (page 76).

● Adjust your diet to suit the time of year (page 67).

Over the next few pages, you will find lists of foods to help you plan a diet to suit your doshas and constitutional type. These suggestions will help you to check the suitability of your present way of eating and make any adjustments as necessary.

Important

The following food guidelines are general recommendations only. They cannot and should not be regarded as a substitute for a detailed, personal diet programme devised by a qualified Ayurvedic practitioner.

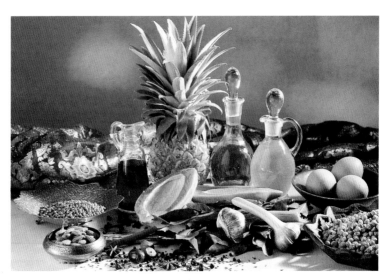

Foods for
vata types

Foods for vata types

Dryness is a characteristic of vata, the "king of the doshas". To achieve their balance, vata types should aim to eat heavy, oily, hot foods. Nourishing stews, baked dishes and soups are among the best kind of meals to pacify vata.

Stews, baked dishes and soups

Rice, pasta, warm milk, cream or freshly baked bread also balance this dosha. On the other hand, cold foods such as salads, raw vegetables or ice-cold drinks intensify vata and should be reduced or avoided.

You should give preference to salty, sour and sweet tastes. Ayurveda also recommends *churnas*, a special seasoning mixture of ground spices which is a highly effective vata pacifier. It achieves the same result taken as a tea either with or after meals.

For vata types prone to irregular digestion, cooked, easily digestible meals help to regulate *agni*, the digestive fire. Since vata types are sensitive to tension, it is especially important that they eat in a calm, pleasant atmosphere.

The following foods are especially good for vata types:

Vegetables and salads: asparagus, beetroot, carrots, cucumber, garlic and onions (not raw), radishes, green beans, sweet potatoes. The following can be eaten in small quantities: potatoes, peas, spinach, courgettes, celery and tomatoes. Boil vegetables and add a little ghee.
Fruit: ripe sweet fruit, such as bananas, apricots, peaches, nectarines, berries, mangoes, honeydew melon, papaya, pineapple, plums, oranges, fresh figs, grapes, grapefruit, lemon and avocado.
Grains: rice, wheat.
Dairy products: all dairy products, especially milk, ghee, cream cheese, butter, yoghurt, cream.
Pulses: chick peas, mung beans, red lentils.
Oils and fats: all cooking oils, especially sesame oil.
Animal products: all kinds of white meat, such as poultry or fish; boiled or scrambled eggs.
Nuts and seeds: all types of nuts and seeds in small quantities, especially almonds.
Sweeteners: natural sweeteners, such as honey, maple syrup, cane sugar products.
Herbs and spices: sweet or warming herbs are specially recommended: aniseed, basil, juniper berries, liquorice, mace, marjoram, caraway, cardamom, green coriander, cinnamon, cloves, cumin, fennel, ginger, bay leaves, black pepper, mustard, nutmeg, oregano, sage, tarragon and thyme.

Vata types should reduce or avoid the following foods:

Vegetables or salads: white or red cabbage, cauliflower; sweet peppers, mushrooms and bean sprouts. In general, vata people have problems digesting raw vegetables and salads.
Fruit: pomegranate, dried fruit, cranberries, pears, unripe fruit, especially bananas.
Grains: millet, maize, barley, buckwheat, rye, oats (uncooked).
Pulses: all pulses, apart from those recommended above.
Sweeteners: honey and white sugar in large quantities.
Meat: red meat, such as beef or pork.

A diet for your constitutional type

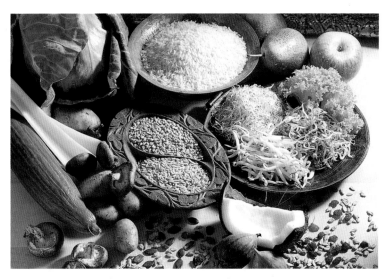

Foods for
pitta types

Food for pitta types

Cool foods

The pitta dosha is hot, which is why people of this constitutional type should eat mainly cool, refreshing foods in summer. Anything that increases heat in the body – such as salt, oil and pungent seasonings – should be reduced or avoided in hot weather.

It is important for pitta types to include some bitter and astringent tastes in their daily diet, which will help to curb their usually hearty appetite. For example, if you eat plenty of green salads, you will be killing two birds with one stone, because salads contain both of these pitta-pacifying *rasas*, in addition to being cold and light.

There are also ground spice mixtures and spiced teas recommended for pitta types. These restore balance and have a beneficial effect on pitta's excessively "fiery" tendencies. Pitta types should make sure they eat regularly and do not skip meals when under stress.

The following foods are especially good for pitta types:

Vegetables and salad: asparagus, broccoli, Brussels sprouts, red and white cabbage, celery, cucumber, green beans, green leaf vegetables, green lettuce, chicory, mushrooms, okra, potatoes, bean sprouts, sweet peppers, courgettes.
Fruit: apples, pineapple, sweet cherries, coconut, figs, grapes, mangoes, lemons, oranges, pears, plums, prunes, raisins, avocados. All fruits should be ripe and sweet.
Grains: barley, oats, wheat, white rice (especially Basmati).
Dairy products: unsalted butter, ghee, cottage cheese, ice cream, milk.
Pulses: green beans, fresh peas, mung beans, chick peas, tofu and other soya products.
Oils and fats: coconut oil, olive oil, soya oil, sunflower oil, ghee.
Animal products: poultry, pheasant, hare, game, egg white.
Nuts and seeds: coconut, sunflower seeds and pumpkin seeds.
Sweeteners: all sweeteners, except honey and molasses.
Herbs and spices: in general, avoid all spices that heat the body too much. The following are permitted in small quantities: cardamom, green coriander, cinnamon, dill, fennel, mint, saffron, turmeric, ginger and black pepper.

Pitta types should reduce or avoid the following foods:

Vegetables and salads: beetroot, carrots, aubergines, radish, tomatoes, chilli peppers, spinach.
Fruit: all sour fruits, such as sour apples, plums, oranges, grapefruit, lemon, morello cherries, cranberries, papaya, peaches, kiwi fruit.
Dairy products: all sour milk products, such as yoghurt, quark, cheese, sour cream, buttermilk.
Grains: millet, maize, buckwheat, rye, brown rice.
Pulses: green lentils (except in soup), red lentils.
Oils and fats: almond oil, sesame oil, corn oil.
Nuts and seeds: sesame seeds, cashew nuts.
Animal products: red meat, such as beef or pork, all seafood, egg yolk.
Spices: all hot spices, such as cayenne pepper, chilli peppers, pepper in large quantities, aniseed, cloves, caraway, mustard seeds, onions, garlic, salt, vinegar, ketchup.

A diet for your constitutional type

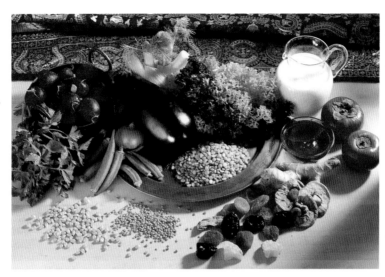

Foods for
kapha types

Foods for kapha types

Light, dry, hot foods

It is difficult to influence the energetic potential of kapha through diet, but poor eating habits over the years can throw this type permanently off balance.

Kapha characteristics are heaviness, oiliness and coldness, so this dosha is increased by heavy, fatty or cold food. If kapha types constantly eat too much, including too many sweet or fatty foods, doshic imbalance is the inevitable result.

On the other hand, everything that is light, dry and hot pacifies kapha. People of this constitutional type should aim to eat low-fat lightly cooked dishes, fresh fruit and raw vegetables. Kapha types can comfortably skip meals, since they are inclined to overeat and easily put on weight.

Pungent, bitter and astringent tastes have a balancing effect on the kapha dosha. In winter, hot and spicy food is advisable, since this helps withstand the cold, damp weather that can upset kapha types. There are also special spice mixtures and blends of tea that pacify kapha (for suppliers see page 92).

The following foods are especially good for kapha types:

Vegetables and salads: most vegetables, including asparagus, broccoli, beetroot, Brussels sprouts, red and white cabbage, cauliflower, carrots, celery, aubergines, garlic, green leaf vegetables, mushrooms, okra, potatoes, bean sprouts, fennel, radish, parsley, all salad leaves, chicory, onions.
Fruit: apples, pears, guavas, pomegranate, cranberries, dates, figs, dried fruits (such as raisins, apricots, figs, prunes).
Grains: barley, buckwheat, maize, millet, rye, white rice in small quantities.
Dairy products: skimmed milk, full-cream milk (in small quantities), buttermilk, ghee (in small quantities).

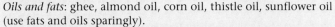

Pulses: all pulses, except soya products and white and black beans.
Oils and fats: ghee, almond oil, corn oil, thistle oil, sunflower oil (use fats and oils sparingly).
Animal products: poultry, prawns, game (in small quantities), scrambled eggs.
Nuts and seeds: sunflower seeds and pumpkin seeds.
Sweeteners: honey
Herbs and spices: all seasonings except salt, especially pungent spices such as ginger, black pepper, coriander, turmeric, cloves, cardamom, cinnamon.

Kapha types should reduce or avoid the following foods:

Vegetables and salads: cucumber, courgettes, pumpkin, sweet potatoes.
Fruit: bananas, sweet grapes, sweet melon, plums, mangoes, coconut, apricots.
Dairy products: cheese, quark, yoghurt, sour milk, cream, full-cream milk and ghee (in large quantities).
Grains: brown rice, oat flakes, wheat or white rice in large quantities.
Nuts and seeds: all nuts.
Sweeteners: sugar, syrup, molasses.
Animal products: seafood (except prawns), beef, pork, lamb.
Spices: salt.

Useful addresses

Ayurveda as an alternative medical therapy is relatively new to this country. However, the proven successes of Ayurvedic herbal treatments are leading to a rapid growth in the popularity of Ayurveda as a therapy. A register of Ayurvedic herbal practitioners and consultants is now in the making. For further information:

Dr Ela Shah
Ayurved Consultancy
50 Elmcroft Crescent
London NW11 9SY
Tel: 0181 455 6598

Dr M S Moorthy
105A Upper Tooting Road
London SW17 7TW
Tel: 0181 682 3876

Index

PICTURE CREDITS
Rainer Schmitz: pages 6/7, 32/33, 35, 36, 37, 38, 44, 45,
46, 47, 48, 49, 50, 51, 52, 53, 54, 55, 57, 70/71, 72, 73,
74, 76, 78, 80, 81, 84, 86, 88, back cover
Photographic styling: Jeanette Heerwager
Michael Nischke: page 66
Fotostudio Teubner: vignette page 77
Marlen Unger-Raabe: front cover , pages 24, 60, 68
Elifie Vierck-Petschelt: graphic page 62

First published by Gräfe und Unzer Verlag GmbH, Munich
© 1995 Gräfe und Unzer
Authorized English language edition published by
Time-Life Books BV, 1066 AZ Amsterdam
© 1997 Time-Life Books BV
First English language printing 1997

English translation by Denise Moseley for
Ros Schwartz Translations, London
Ayurvedic consultant: Dr Ela Shah
Editor: Christine Noble
Layout and DTP: Dawn McGinn

ISBN 0 7054 3531 8

20 19 18 17 16 15 14 13 12 11 10 9 8 7 6 5 4 3 2 1

About this book

Ayurveda is a system of holistic healing which originated in India thousands of years ago. The name is derived from the Sanskrit *ved*, meaning knowledge or science, and *ayu*, daily life or life cycle. Ayurveda is concerned with every aspect of human life: mind, body, behaviour and environment. As a system of healing it concentrates on preserving well-being and on improving our spiritual, intellectual and physical ability to heal ourselves. Guided by Ayurvedic teachings, we can learn to recognize and treat problems caused by diet or stress, and how to avoid them in the future. This book provides a brief introduction to the principles of Ayurvedic healing. Through a detailed questionnaire it enables you to determine your constitutional type according to Ayurveda. It then explains how you can incorporate Ayurvedic practice into your daily life through Yoga and breathing exercises, massage, aromatherapy and colour therapy, and last but not least, diet.

About the author

Karen Schutt was born in 1955 in Freidberg, Hessen, Germany, and graduated in communication sciences, psychology and education. A freelance writer since 1985, she has published numerous books, mainly dealing with health matters.

About the general consultant

Dr George Lewith is one of the UK's leading practitioners, researchers and writers in the field of complementary medicine. After training in conventional medicine, he spent four years as a physician in major London hospitals before deciding to dedicate his time to complementary practice. He studied acupuncture at the College of Traditional Chinese Medicine in Nanking and was co-founder of the Centre for the Study of Complementary Medicine, which practices in Southampton and Harley Street offering many alternative therapies. Dr Lewith also heads a research unit at Southampton University's School of Medicine conducting clinical studies into the effectiveness of complementary medical treatments.

Titles in this series